Laparoscopy in Urology

MALCOLM J. COPTCOAT
ChM FRCS (Urol)
Consultant Urologist and Director of Surgery
King's College Hospital, London

AND

ADRIAN D. JOYCE
MS FRCS (Urol)
Consultant Urologist
Leeds General Infirmary

OXFORD
BLACKWELL SCIENTIFIC PUBLICATIONS
LONDON EDINBURGH BOSTON
MELBOURNE PARIS BERLIN VIENNA

Dedicated to John (*mentor meus*)

Editorial Offices:
Osney Mead, Oxford OX2 0EL
25 John Street, London WC1N 2BL
23 Ainslie Place, Edinburgh EH3 6AJ
238 Main Street, Cambridge
Massachusetts 02142, USA
54 University Street, Carlton
Victoria 3053, Australia

Other Editorial Offices:
Librairie Arnette SA
1, rue de Lille
75007 Paris
France

Blackwell Wissenschafts-Verlag GmbH
Düsseldorfer Str. 38
D-10707 Berlin
Germany

Blackwell MZV
Feldgasse 13
A-1238 Wien
Austria

First published 1994

Set by DSM, Oxford
Printed and bound in Great Britain
at the the University Press, Cambridge

DISTRIBUTORS
Marston Book Services Ltd
PO Box 87
Oxford OX2 0DT
(*Orders*: Tel: 0865 791155
Fax: 0865 791927
Telex: 837515)

USA
Blackwell Scientific Publications, Inc.
238 Main Street
Cambridge, MA 02142
(*Orders*: Tel: 800 759-6102
617 876-7000)

Canada
Times Mirror Professional Publishing, Ltd
130 Flaska Drive
Markham, Ontario L6G 1B8
(*Orders*: Tel: 800 268-4178
416 470-6739)

Australia
Blackwell Scientific Publications Pty Ltd
54 University Street
Carlton, Victoria 3053
(*Orders*: Tel: 03 347-5552)

A catalogue record for this title
is available from the British Library

ISBN 0-86542-814-X

Library of Congress
Cataloging-in-Publication data

Laparoscopy in Urology/
by Malcolm J. Coptcoat and Adrian D.
Joyce.
p. cm.
Includes bibliographic references
and index.
ISBN 0-86542-814-X
1. Genitourinary organs—Surgery.
2. Laparoscopic surgery.
I. Coptcoat, Malcolm J.
II. Joyce, Adrian D.
[DNLM: 1. Laparoscopy—methods.
2. Surgery, Laparoscopic.
3. Urinary tract—surgery.
WJ 168 L2995 1994]
RD571.L36 1994
617.4'6059—dc20
DNLM/DLC
for Library of Congress

Contents

List of Contributors

PAUL CARTER MD FRCS
Senior Urological Registrar, King's College Hospital, Denmark Hill, London SE5 9RS, England

MALCOLM J. COPTCOAT ChM FRCS (Urol)
Consultant Urologist and Director of Surgery, King's College Hospital, Denmark Hill, London SE5 9RS, England

CHRISTOPHER G. EDEN MB BS FRCS
Wickham Fellow and Honorary Urological Registrar, King's College Hospital, Denmark Hill, London SE5 9RS, England

DAVID GREEN FRC Anaes
Consultant Anaesthetist, King's College Hospital, Denmark Hill, London SE5 9RS, England

ADRIAN D. JOYCE MS FRCS (Urol)
Consultant Urologist, Leeds General Infirmary, Great George Street, Leeds LS1 3EX, England

MARCIN MATUSZEWSKI MD
Resident in Urology and Visiting Fellow to King's College Hospital, Medical Academy, Kieturakisa 1, Gdansk, Poland

ANGUS MITCHELL FRC Anaes
Senior Anaesthetic Registrar, King's College Hospital, Denmark Hill, London SE5 9RS, England

Preface

Surgical practice is undergoing a revolution. Minimally invasive techniques are rapidly replacing traditional open surgical procedures. The epitome of the change is to be found in laparoscopy.

In 1990, laparoscopy in urology was confined to diagnosis of the intra-abdominal testicle. Many of us had witnessed the complex operative gynaecological laparoscopy of Professor Kurt Semm but were frustrated by a lack of the instrumentation needed in urology. However, an explosion in the use of laparoscopic cholecystectomy has now not only changed general surgery but led to the innovative developments in equipment that allow us to perform complex laparoscopic procedures in urology.

Laparoscopy is a team effort, and the establishment of a laparoscopic centre of excellence in King's College Hospital has been possible only through the support and skills of my surgical and nursing colleagues. Innovations in surgery in this decade may spring from an individual but are clarified and modified very quickly by the wider international team. I am especially indebted to Ralph Clayman, Howard Winfield, Lou Kavoussi and many others who have made unselfish and forthcoming contributions to our pooled practical knowledge of laparoscopy in urology.

Acknowledgements

I am indebted to my Personal Assistant, Susan Horrell, for her invaluable assistance in preparing this book. Chris Eden and I took the photographs.

M.J.C.

1: Introduction

M.J. COPTCOAT AND A.D. JOYCE

Lord Lister's portrait hangs in the consultants' room at King's College Hospital, London. His pioneering work with aseptic techniques and his introduction of general anaesthesia to British surgery have made him one of the pillars of surgical wisdom in Great Britain. His solemn features give no hint to the exciting frontiers that his work opened up for surgeons who followed him. Just over 100 years ago he is quoted as saying 'These are exciting times to be a surgeon.' There is obviously a double peak to this excitement with the explosion of endoscopic and, in particular, laparoscopic surgery.

Endoscopic surgery is rapidly becoming a popular alternative to traditional operative open procedures for a variety of diseases. Laparoscopic biliary tract surgery, laparoscopic appendicectomy, laparoscopic gynaecological procedures, laparoscopic urological procedures, the thoracoscopic treatment of pneumothorax and persistent pleural effusions as well as arthroscopic examination and treatment of joint spaces have all become accepted endoscopic procedures. If conducted safely, endoscopic surgery offers savings in total health care as a result of short hospital stays and a more rapid return to normal activities. These are factors that are appealing to commercial health-care providers and the public themselves. There is now an increased public awareness that endoscopic surgery is associated with less pain and less cosmetic disfigurement. This is exemplified by the recent overwhelming introduction of laparoscopic cholecystectomy, which had attracted only minor curiosity when it was first performed in 1987. The exponential acceptance of this procedure has been stimulated by patient demands.

Many of us may not wish to learn new procedures when we have been in practice for a number of years but more than ever before our personal preference for a particular procedure is going to be overhauled by current health education and patients' new expectations.

There is a disadvantage for state health care providers such as the National Health Service with the advent of endoscopic surgery. The capital outlay costs and minimal disposable costs of this type of surgery can probably be written into future budget plans. But the impact on theatre time and expertise will cause large repercussions in the way we structure our current surgical practice. Many of these endoscopic procedures take up to twice as long as their open counterparts. The ultimate advantages are not in question but at present there is not the operating time, theatre personnel or surgical expertise available to introduce this revolution suddenly. These are important

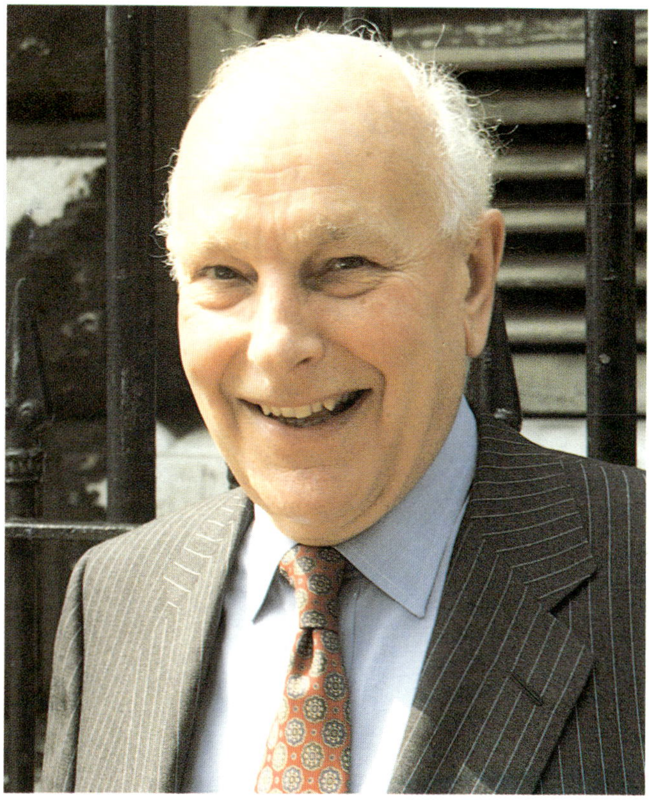

Fig. 1.1 Mr John Wickham, London, England: endoscopic pioneer and founder of the Minimally Invasive Therapy Society.

matters that must be addressed in the way we plan our departments and train our surgeons in the future. These horizons have been anticipated by only a few and no one stands out more than John Wickham (Fig. 1.1). Any difficulties that we might have in introducing these procedures to our hospitals can be blamed partly upon our lack of trust in this man's visionary thinking in the past. The formation of the Minimally Invasive Therapy Society and its close association with both industry and health-care economists will go a long way towards bringing these changes about.

Laparoscopy is transforming general surgery and general surgeons. The same revolution is going to occur in urology, and for once we have sat on our high-technology, minimally invasive laurels for a little too long.

Laparoscopy has previously been regarded as an interesting clinical diagnostic tool with very few applications. It has been well documented that laparoscopy could be helpful in localizing the impalpable undescended testicle when both ultrasound and computerized tomography (CT) have failed to help. But the numbers of these cases that an individual urologist sees are small and so the technique of laparoscopy has been left very much in the background. Laparoscopy need not be merely diagnostic. Here is a list of the operative laparoscopic procedures currently being performed in the urology department of King's College Hospital:

Laparoscopic abdominal orchidectomy
Laparoscopic abdominal orchidopexy (first stage)
Laparoscopic varicocelectomy
Laparoscopic inguinal herniorrhaphy
Laparoscopic appendicectomy
Laparoscopic pelvic lymphadenectomy
Laparoscopic para-aortic lymphadenectomy
Laparoscopic retroperitoneal surgery
- (a) Ureterolysis
- (b) Ureterolithotomy
- (c) Deroofing renal cyst
- (d) Nephrectomy
- (e) Pyeloplasty

Laparoscopic transperitoneal nephrectomy
- (a) Simple
- (b) Radical
- (c) Nephroureterectomy

Laparoscopic colposuspension
Laparoscopic bladder transsection
Laparoscopic ileal conduit diversion
Laparoscopic partial cystectomy
Laparoscopic lymphocele drainage

Many urologists may consider that whilst it might be feasible to carry out all of these procedures using a laparoscope, it will not be without a great deal of operative time and technology overlay. This perception is not justified.

One must return to the patient-priority concept of minimally invasive therapy (Wickham 1987), and that is to achieve the ideal operative result with minimal trauma and a rapid return to normal activities for the patient. This is witnessed in King's College Hospital when a postoperative laparoscopic nephrectomy case requires only oral analgesics, is able to tolerate an oral diet on the first operative day and goes home on the second postoperative day.

The above list of laparoscopic procedures is just a snapshot in the evolution of minimally invasive surgery, however. There have been three evolutionary steps so far. First, diagnosis; second, minor surgical techniques such as biopsy, clipping, cutting and, third, removal of large tissue volumes, such as a nephrectomy or splenectomy. The currently developing fourth step is that of laparoscopic reconstruction. Reconstruction, or rather the specific technique of tissue anastomosis, requires the re-evaluation of alternative technology such as glues, laser welding and absorbable stapling devices, because laparoscopic suturing is not just difficult to master but often inappropriate when working in a confined space. In a solution to this problem, we begin to see the divergence of laparoscopy from a method of merely copying open procedures. This will blossom when surgeons can rationalize the advantages that laparoscopy brings. Although a reduction in the trauma of access brings obvious advantages, there comes a point when the complexity of the intra-abdominal procedure produces greater potential morbidity. Thus, the internal part of our laparoscopic procedures must be more refined. Until this happens, the rationale for carrying out a laparoscopic radical cystectomy or prostatectomy will be based on feasibility for the surgeon and not decreased morbidity for the patient. The laparoscope is an internal operating microscope, and the dissection and manipulation should be precise. Our instrumentation does not yet always allow that, but it will come and with it the fifth evolutionary step of laparoscopy.

This book will undoubtedly age very rapidly. But during its short life span, we hope that it will serve as a practical guide to urologists wishing to take on operative laparoscopy. None of these procedures will by themselves be performed very frequently in a department but the increasing spectrum will allow experience to be gained and applied for any of them.

Reference

Wickham J.E.A. (1987) The 'new surgery'. *British Medical Journal*, **295**, 1581–2.

2: History of Laparoscopy

M.J. COPTCOAT AND M. MATUSZEWSKI

Laparoscopy is very much a development of the twentieth century. Kelling (1901) described a case report of inspection of the abdominal cavity of a dog using a Nitze cystoscope introduced through a small stab wound. The same author then described his use of this laparoscopic technique in man in 1923. Ott (1901) in Petrograd (now St Petersburg) described an alternative method for inspection of the abdominal contents by making a small incision and looking inside with a head mirror and indirect illumination. Ott called this technique 'ventroscopy'.

The father of what we now regard as laparoscopy, and indeed the first to use the term 'laparoscopy', was Jacobeus in Stockholm. In fact, 'laparo-' is literally translated from the Greek as 'flank', a combining form denoting a relationship to the loin or flank and sometimes used loosely in reference to the abdomen. This would not be the only instance when the most popular name has quite rightly its origin in a pioneer's technique rather than from a true etymological source. Jacobeus (1910) reported the use of a cystoscope for examination of both the peritoneal and pleural cavities. His instrument was inserted through a sheath trocar system. Both water and air were used for distention of the cavity, but the indication for the majority of his early patients was that of ascites when a concomitant paracentesis could be performed.

Little thought had been given at this time to the artificial introduction of air or water to increase the peritoneal cavity's dimensions. Bernheim (1911) from the Johns Hopkins Hospital in Baltimore called his technique of abdominal inspection 'organoscopy'. He utilized a proctoscope and was the first to state that the presence of ascites was not necessary. He used air for insufflation. He described two cases. One was referred by another famous surgeon, Halstead, with a pancreatic tumour. The organoscopy was carried out to look for metastases. None were identified, and in the true spirit of validation, they then proceeded to an open exploration to confirm the findings. They had been correct. A second case was described of a patient who presented with an acute abdomen for whom a provisional diagnosis of a gastric ulcer had been made. Acute appendicitis was identified during organoscopy and the patient subsequently underwent a successful appendicectomy, albeit by open incision. It is a little embarrassing to realize that the use of abdominal endoscopic inspection for the acute abdomen had been described in 1911 and we still find that many surgeons have not realized its potential in 1993 in this clinical situation.

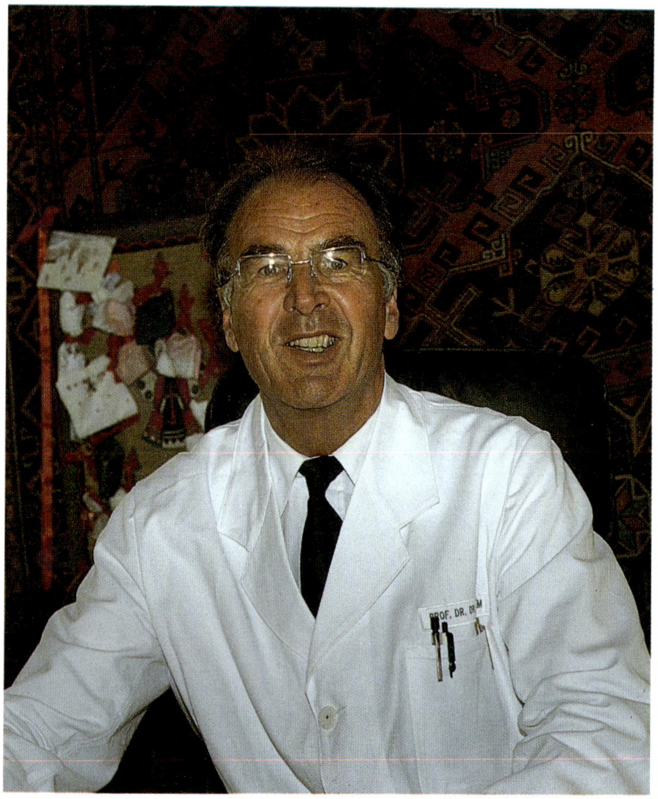

Fig. 2.1 Professor Kurt Semm, Kiel, Germany. The pioneer of operative laparoscopy in gynaecology. He also performed the first laparoscopic appendicectomy.

Nordentöft (1912) was the first to introduce a sharp-pointed trocar to ease the introduction of the sheath. At the same time, he advocated the use of the head-down or Trendelenberg position to make the insertion of the trocar and cannula safer.

Stolkind (1919) popularized the use of the laparoscope and made several innovative steps. He was the first to introduce the use of a smaller sharp cannula into the abdomen, through which air could be insufflated. This was then followed by the larger sharp-pointed trocar and cannula that would take the telescope. Zollikofer (1925) introduced the concept of carbon dioxide for insufflation, remarking that it was much safer than air, but not really going into great details as to why at this stage. With laparoscopy established as a safe diagnostic procedure, and with the instrumentation and technique accepted by most physicians and surgeons, we turn to Fervers (1933), who was the first to carry out some form of operative procedure. He described the technique of adhesiolysis. For this, he required the introduction of a second port for the insertion of scissors.

A very interesting contribution was made by Ruddock (1937) who reported on a series of 200 patients. He began the argument that has been taken up more recently regarding the economics of laparoscopy. He showed quite clearly that the decreased morbidity in his patients who were saved from open surgery easily outweighed the slight increase in cost of the laparoscopic procedure itself. This was a very detailed paper. Forty-nine of his procedures were for biopsy of intra-abdominal malignancies. Not only was he well ahead of his time in terms of health economics, he was also a physician already moving in on his colleagues' surgical domain. Does this have an echo in the present time? Veress (1938), an innovative surgeon from Hungary, introduced the spring-loaded insufflation needle which is little different from the one we use routinely today. Further changes in laparoscopy were slow to be reported, probably because of the continued criticism by fellow physicians and surgeons.

The controlled automatic insufflator was introduced by Semm (Fig. 2.1) in the late 1960s, and it is Semm himself (1978, 1982a, 1982b, 1983, 1986, 1989) who began to describe the more elaborate operative procedures that most of the gynaecological world seemed to choose to ignore until the late 1980s. It is interesting to see that Semm's work, which also included the first reported laparoscopic appendicectomy (Semm 1983), once heavily criticized even by gynaecologists and general surgeons in Germany, has now received a fresh appraisal. As a living father of this technology, his presence is in even greater demand around the world.

However, the catalyst for the explosion of interest in operative laparoscopy focuses on the laparoscopic cholecystectomy. This was first reported by Dubois *et al.* (1989) who then went on to describe three years of experience of this technique in 1990. On the other side of the Atlantic, Reddick *et al.* (1989) reported on his series of over 200 laparoscopic cholecystectomies when most other surgeons were still arguing over the theoretical advantages. Reddick began to convince his colleagues, and more importantly the public, that laparoscopic techniques were the way ahead.

It is difficult to understand the very rapid acceptance of these techniques by both clinicians and patients in the last five years, but it probably reflects improved communication and health education. As a prime example of minimally invasive surgery, laparoscopy not only benefits the patient in terms of a more rapid return to normal activities and reduced morbidity but also benefits those who control our health economy. There has been an undeniable interest from government officials, hospital administrators and politicians in such techniques and this has again reinforced the public's awareness. What has been in the melting pot for 92 years has now snowballed with rapidly gaining momentum, and each new publication from each newly formed journal brings yet another innovative step to refine further the techniques of laparoscopy and expand its horizons.

Several urologists have been involved in the development of laparoscopy in the last 10 years. Eshghi *et al.* (1985) described a percutaneous transperitoneal laparoscopic approach to a pelvic kidney and subsequent endoscopic removal of a staghorn calculus. Das & Amar (1988) and Whitfield & Ryan (1990) also discussed the potential for

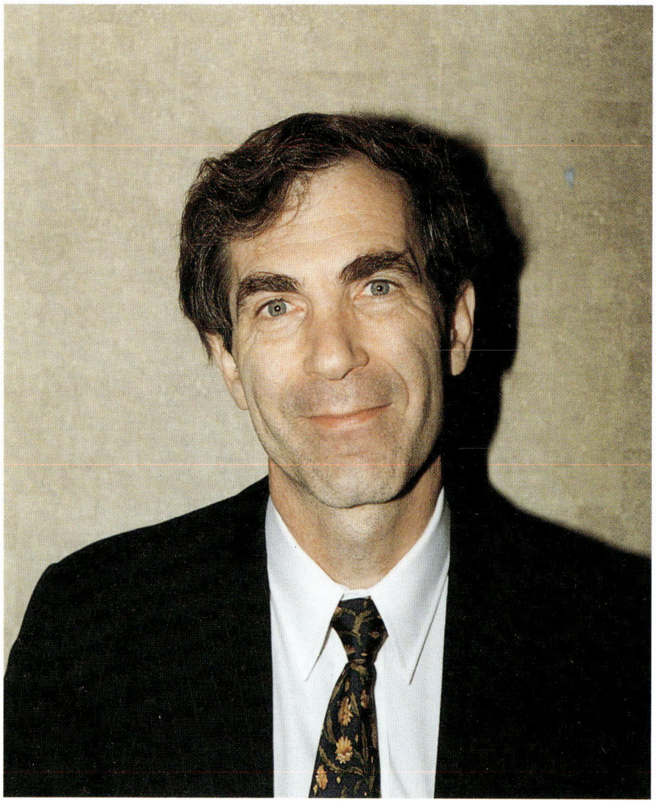

Fig. 2.2 Professor Ralph Clayman, St Louis, USA. In 1991 he performed the first laparoscopic nephrectomy.

laparoscopic techniques in urology, but the greatest credit must always go to Ralph Clayman (Fig. 2.2), who not has only made enormous contributions to endourology as a whole, but developed many of the more complicated techniques such as a laparoscopic nephrectomy (Clayman *et al.* 1991), and then convinced the rest of us that this was the way ahead.

References

Bernheim B.M. (1911) Organoscopy: Cystoscopy of the abdominal cavity. *Annals of Surgery*, **53**, 764.

Clayman R., Kavoussi L., Soper N. *et al.* (1991) Laparoscopic nephrectomy: Initial case report. *Journal of Urology*, **146**, 278–82.

Das S. & Amar A.D. The impact of laparoscopy on modern urological practice. *Urological Clinics of North America*, **15**: 3, 537–40.

Dubois F., Berthelot G., Levard H. (1989) Cholecystectomie par coelioscopie. *Nouvelle presse médicale*, **18**, 980–2.

Dubois F., Icard P., Berthelot G., Levard H. (1990) Coelioscopic cholecystectomy. *Annals of Surgery*, **211**, 60–2.

Eshghi A.M., Roth J.S., Smith A.D. (1985) Percutaneous transperitoneal approach to a pelvic kidney for endourological removal of a staghorn calculus. *Journal of Urology*, **134**, 525–7.

Fervers C. (1933) Die Laparoskopie mit dem Zystokope. Ein Beitrag zur Vereinfachung der Technik und zur endoskopischen Strangdurchtrennung in der Bauchole. *Medizinische Klinik*, **29**, 1042–5.

Jacobeus H.C. (1910) Über die Möglichkeiten, die Zystoskopie bei Untersuchung seroser Hohlungen anzuwenden. *Münchener medezinische Wochenschrift*, **57**, 2090–2.

Kelling G. (1901) Über Ösophagoskopie, Gastroskopie und Colioskopie. *Münchener medezinische Wochenschrift*, **49**, 21–4.

Nordentöft S. (1912) Über Endoskopie geschlossener Kavitaten mittels meines Trokar-Endoskopes. *Verhandlungen der Deutchen Gesellschaft für Gynakologie*, **41**, 78-81.

Ott D. (1901) Illumination of the abdomen (ventroscopia) (Russian). *Journal Akusche-zologii Zhenskoi*, **15**, 1045.

Reddick E.J., Olsen D., Daniell J., Saye W. *et al.* (1989) Laparoscopic laser cholecystectomy. *Lasers in Medicine and Surgery*, February, 38–40.

Ruddock J.C. (1937) Peritoneoscopy. *Surgery, Gynaecology and Obstetrics*, **65**, 623.

Semm K. (1978) Tissue puncher and loop ligation. New aids for surgical therapeutic pelviscopy (laparoscopy): Endoscopic intra-abdominal surgery. *Endoscopy*, **10**, 119–27.

Semm K. (1982a) Advances in pelviscopic surgery (appendicectomy) *Current Problems in Obstetrics, Gynaecology and Fertility*, **5** (10).

Semm K. (1982b) The endoscopic intra-abdominal suture. *Geburtshilfe und Frauenheilkunde*, **42**, 56–7.

Semm K. (1983) Endoscopic appendicectomy. *Endoscopy*, **15**, 59–64.

Semm K. (1986) Operative pelviscopy. *British Medical Bulletin*, **42**, 284–95.

Semm K. (1989) History. In: *Operative Gynaecologic Endoscopy* (eds J.S. Sanfillipo & R.L. Levine). Springer-Verlag, New York.

Stolkind E.J. (1919) The value of pleuroscopy (thoracoscopy) in the diagnosis of pulmonary diseases and laparoscopy in the diagnosis of abdominal diseases. *The Medical Press*, 1 January.

Veress J. (1938) Neues Instrument zur Ausführung von Brust oder Bauchpunktionen. *Deutsche medizinische Wochenschrift*, 41, 1480–1.

Whitfield H.N., Ryan K.J. (1990) Experimental laparoscopic surgery: potential clinical applications in urology. *Journal of Endourology*, **4**: 1, 37–47.

Zollikofer R. (1925) Zur Laparoskopie. *Schweizerische medizinische Wochenschrift*, **5**, 264–5.

3: Instrumentation

M.J. COPTCOAT AND C.G. EDEN

Telescopes

One of the most significant advances in rigid endoscopy was the development of the rod lens system in 1966 by the British optical physicist Hopkins. His design, which utilizes air spaces for the lenses, resulted in vastly improved image brightness and clarity. Most of the endoscope manufacturers now use a hybrid of this system, and contrary to popular opinion amongst urologists, there is a great deal of difference between the different manufacturers' telescopes. The rigid endoscope consists of an objective lens, relay lens, eye piece lens and illumination light guide. The eye piece lens has an approximate magnification of x 3 and this could be easily increased for future endoscopic microsurgical work.

The field of view varies with each manufacturer's endoscope. The 'field of view' describes the area observable from the tip of the endoscope. The greater the field of view, the greater the area that can be observed, given that the distance from the lens is the same. If the visual field is merely widened, the image will become smaller. The 'observed field of view' refers to the size of the visual field observed through the rigid endoscope, thus the larger the observed field of view, the larger the image (Fig. 3.1). The 'direction of view' (Fig. 3.2) refers to the angle between the centre of the visual field and the longitudinal axis of the endoscope. Standard laparoscopes have a 0° or 30°

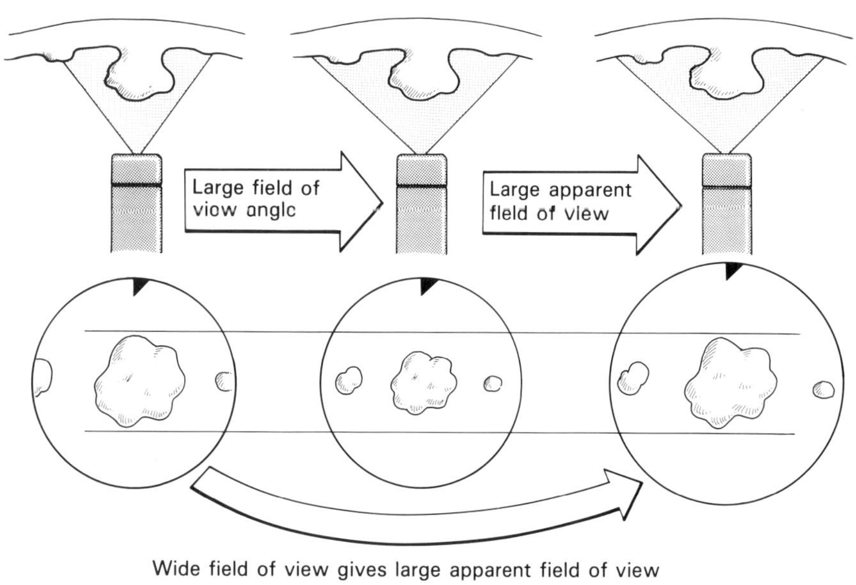

Fig. 3.1 Field of view and apparent field of view in rigid laparoscopes vary with each manufacturer's endoscope. The greater the field of view, the greater the area that can be observed. If the visual field is merely widened, the image will become smaller. The larger the 'observed field of view', the larger the image.

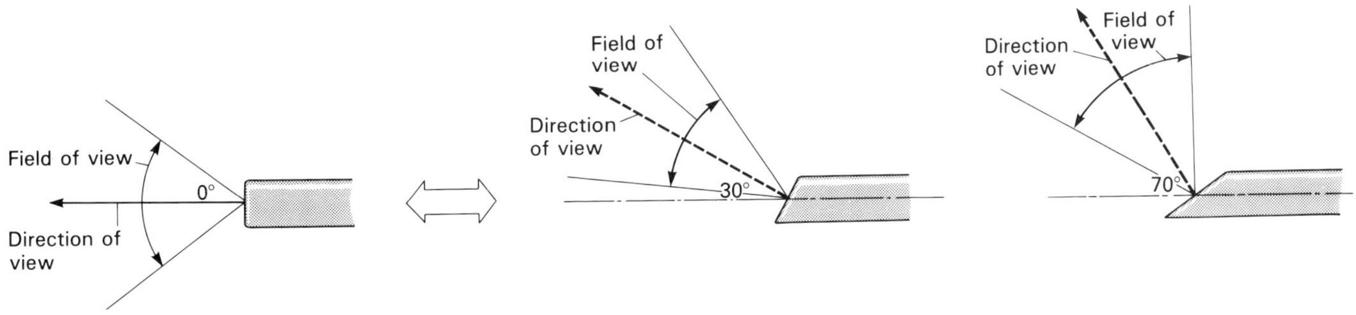

Fig. 3.2 Direction of view and field of view of a laparoscope. The 'direction of view' refers to the angle between the centre of the visual field and the longitudinal axis of the endoscope.

direction of view but we will probably see the introduction of increased angles for specific complex manoeuvres. Endoscopic instrument orientation is easiest when visualized through a 0° telescope but one sometimes has a restricted view of the site of dissection and a different direction of view can help the operator to see over obstacles. The disadvantage in instrument orientation is then of secondary importance.

The overall diameter of the telescopes used in laparoscopy is approximately 9 mm and they require a 10 mm port. Telescopes are available with an integrated working channel. The presence of such a working channel usually reduces the diameter and therefore the clarity of the lens image, and using manipulative devices in this way is usually confined to simple manoeuvres such as the clipping of Fallopian tubes. They do not really have a place in more complex operative laparoscopy where more sensitive instrument orientation is required.

One of the greatest practical problems during prolonged operative laparoscopy is misting of the objective lens within the abdomen. This occurs because of the relative imbalance between intraperitoneal temperatures and the temperature of the telescope. It is exacerbated by the use of diathermy or lasers near the lens.

Up until now, the only ways to deal with this have been the repeated removal and warming of the telescope in hot water or the use of demisting solutions. Even the latter solution requires removal of the telescope every 10–15 minutes. This can be very tedious during a complex manoeuvre. Some manufacturers have recently introduced a telescope with its own irrigating and self-cleaning lens. Whilst this has added bulk to the telescope it has proved to be one way around an otherwise irritating problem.

Cameras

Coptcoat spent some time with Professor Semm in Kiel, Germany, in 1988. Semm had been carrying out operative laparoscopy since 1973, and 97% of his routine gynaecological workload was then carried out

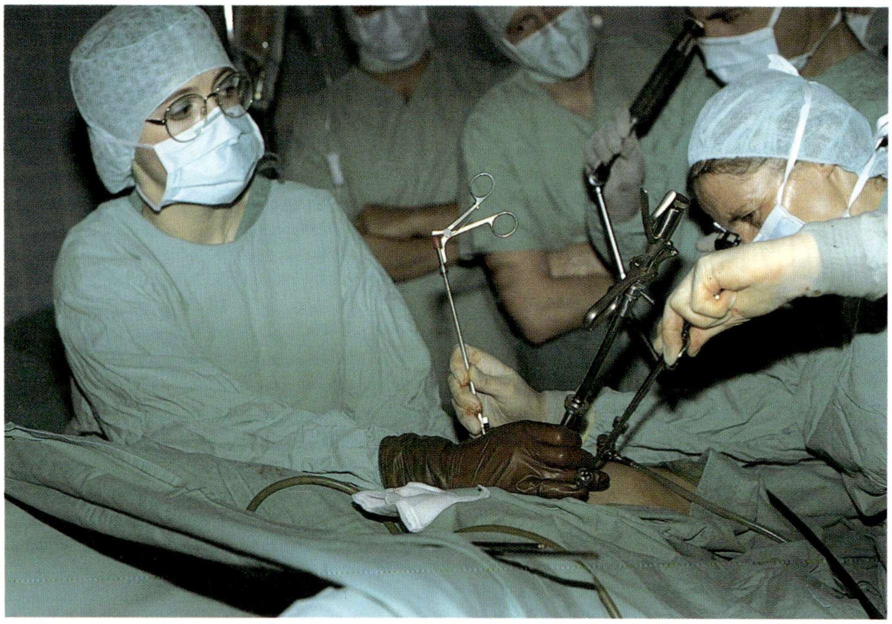

Fig 3.3 Complex operative laparoscopy in Kiel in 1989, without the benefit of the video camera.

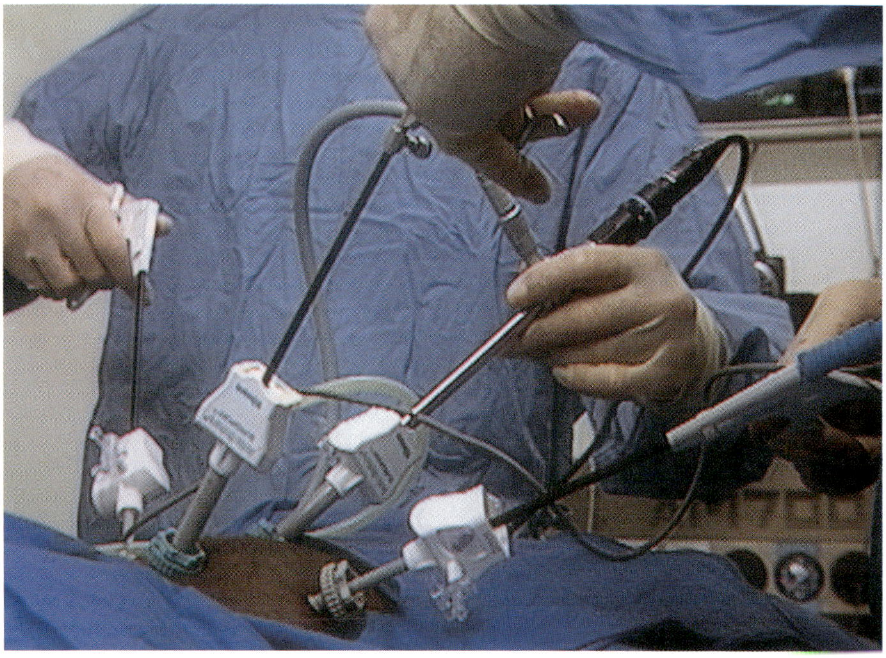

Fig 3.4 Complex operative laparoscopy in London in 1993.

laparoscopically. Coptcoat was able to witness the need for multiple theatres because of the increased operative time, but one small observation stood out more than the rest and this was the requirement of gymnastic qualities by the primary operators (Fig. 3.3).

At this time, video cameras were not in use and the operator had to keep his or her eye close to the telescope whilst moving instruments at full arm's length. Whilst one is welcome to carry on in this way, the advent of laparoscopic cholecystectomy performed using the video camera has introduced an indirect and ergonomically more

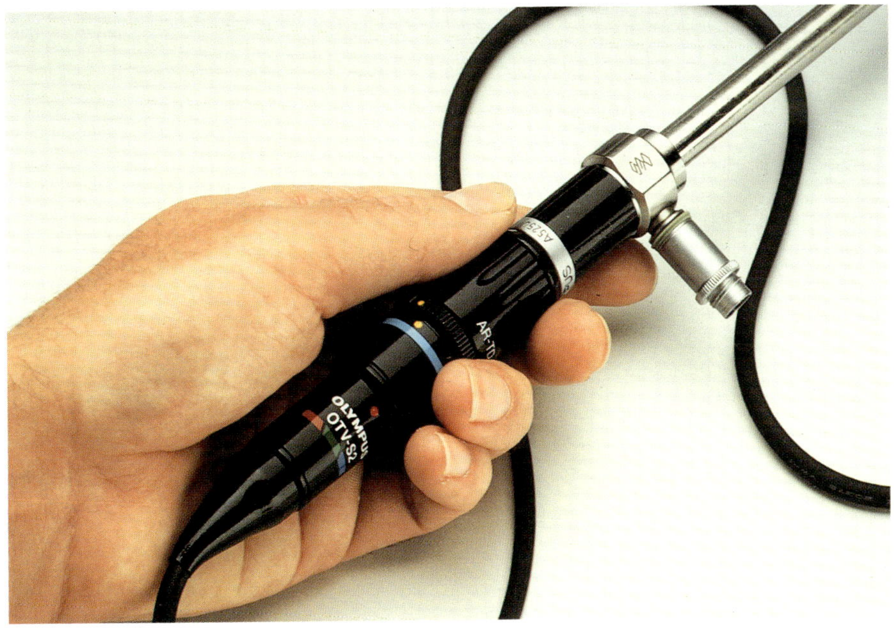

Fig. 3.5 A high-quality CCD camera used for operative laparoscopy.

Table 3.1 Imaging systems tested at King's College Hospital, London

Camera	Light source	Telescope
GU-8001	8003	8011
Olympus OTV-S2	CLV-10	A5254A
Olympus OTV-S4	CLV-10	A5254A
Storz 9050PB	450DV	26033AP
Wolf 5500.11	5130	8934.441

pleasing type of surgery to most of our departments. Operating whilst watching a video monitor (Fig. 3.4) is a new and initially demanding experience with its own learning curve. However, most of us as urologists should be familiar with this if we are carrying out our prostatic resections in a similar way.

The modern charge-coupled device (CCD) camera (Fig. 3.5) is an essential requirement for teaching and training and its routine use will allow us to make the step into operative laparoscopy with much less difficulty. The camera should be handed to a urologist whenever any form of endoscopy is taking place.

There are many CCD cameras on the market at present, and we have carried out an objective assessment of five of these systems. The optical design and image quality were assessed using an optical bench, a Sony UP5000 colour videoprinter and three test cards. Vertical, horizontal and rotational scales on the optical bench were set to zero before the telescope was clamped in position with its window 45 mm from the test target.

The light source output was set to automatic and the image was colour-balanced. The target was manually focused using the central part of the test grid (KeyMed 1992). Each set of videoprints was examined by an independent optical engineer without knowledge of the corresponding imaging system and was assessed with regard to optical design, image quality, illumination and colour rendition.

There was a surprisingly large and dramatic difference in the optical performance of the imaging systems tested. Whilst the performance of some was disappointing, two of these systems produced images with excellent resolution, brightness and colour rendition: the GU-8001 camera, 8003 light source and 8011 telescope; and the Olympus OTV-S4 camera, CLV-10 light source and A5254A telescope combination.

Of the two, the GU system produced an image with considerable distortion, field curvature and moderate astigmatism, whereas the Olympus system produced a flat image with no distortion and only very slight astigmatism.

The optics of the Olympus OTV-S4 CCD camera, when used with the CLV-10 light source and A5254A telescope, are superior to the other systems tested and provide an image with good resolution, brightness and colour rendition. Interestingly, only the two Olympus systems produced an image free of distortion or field curvature and with very slight astigmatism. This is clearly a great asset in operative laparoscopy, in which depth perception is always difficult because of the two-dimensional image provided.

The other significant visual handicap in operative laparoscopy is the left-to-right inverted image on the first assistant's monitor when two monitors are being used, as in a laparoscopic nephrectomy. Great patience on the part of the operator and careful practice on the part of the assistant are necessary!

Current developments in CCD technology include improved light sensitivity (increased pixels), better colour rendition (three-chip cameras) and the use of three-dimensional imaging systems. 3-D cameras are now available but are very bulky and expensive; we all eagerly await their refinement because of the dramatic effect it will have on our endocoordination.

The routine use of an imaging system in endourology (O'Boyle 1990) reduces the possibility of contact with potentially contaminated body fluids, fatigue and, ultimately, operating time. It increases image size, accuracy and comfort as well as interest in the operation by theatre staff and is also an ideal teaching aid. Its routine use in endourology enables the neolaparoscopist to improve endocoordination and orientation before embarking on operative laparoscopy with which he will then rapidy become comfortable.

Insufflators

The artificial space within the peritoneal cavity is achieved and maintained by filling with a gas that distends the abdominal wall. This is termed the pneumoperitoneum.

In the history of laparoscopy, many gases have been used for establishing a pneumoperitoneum, including room air, nitrous oxide, oxygen and carbon dioxide. Air and oxygen create a higher risk in terms of air embolism. In addition, they support combustion, which is dangerous when using electrocautery or laser energy. Nitrous oxide has unpredictable effects because of its rapid absorption into the blood stream. Nitrous oxide was commonly used for diagnostic laparoscopy but because the gas also supports combustion, its use tends to preclude any dissection.

Carbon dioxide has therefore become the standard gas used for creating a pneumoperitoneum. It is relatively safe in that it can be injected directly into the blood stream in volumes up to 100 ml per minute without serious metabolic effects. It also suppresses combustion. This is all very fortunate because carbon dioxide is also the most readily available and inexpensive gas.

A modern insufflator (see Fig. 3.6) is now a piece of sophisticated equipment that has been developed to deliver carbon dioxide automatically from a high-pressured pressure tank through a regulator and into the patient at predetermined flow rates. These machines constantly monitor the intra-abdominal pressure and stop the flow once a certain pressure is reached.

They usually indicate the rate of flow and record the total volume of gas delivered from the machine. Rapid insufflation into the abdomen is necessary when there is a leak around a valve or during the exchange of instruments. Therefore, operative laparoscopic surgery requires a high-flow insufflator capable of delivering at least 6 l of gas per minute. The new machines are set with an upper pressure limit of 15 mm of mercury. It is safer to work at a pressure of 10 mm of mercury during procedures that last several hours. A lower

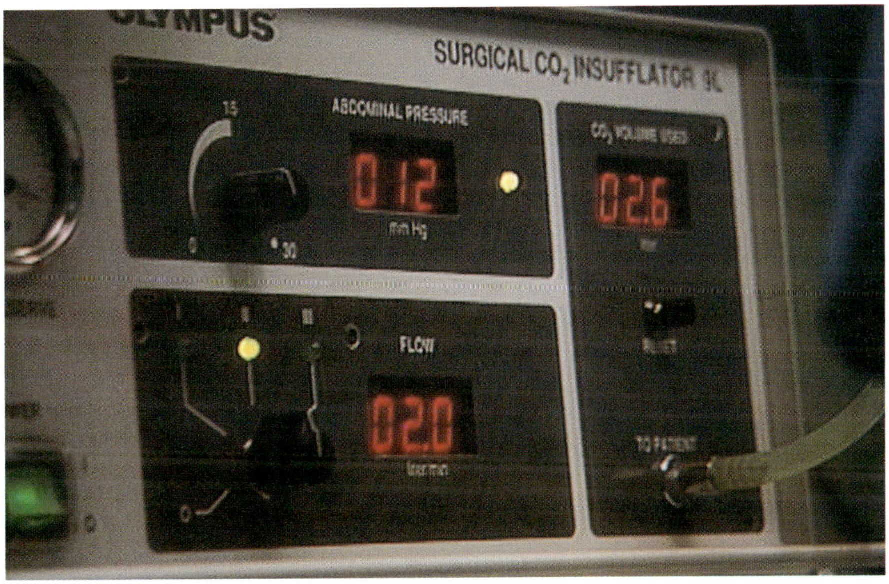

Fig 3.6 A modern, automatic high-flow carbon dioxide insufflator used in operative laparoscopy.

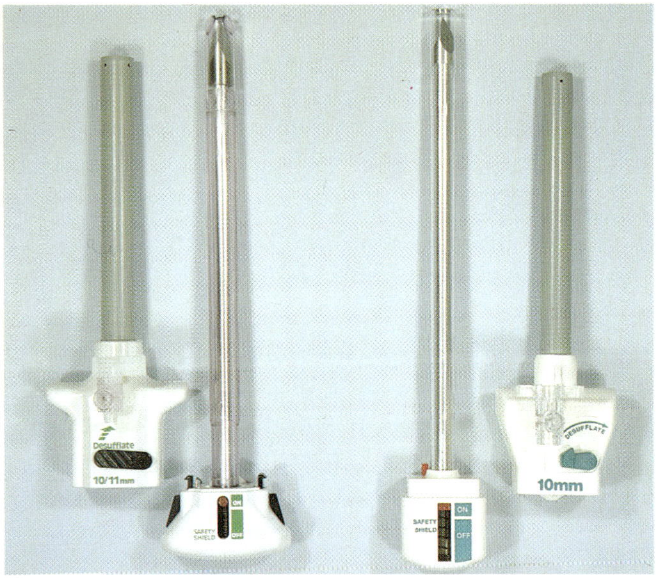

Fig. 3.7

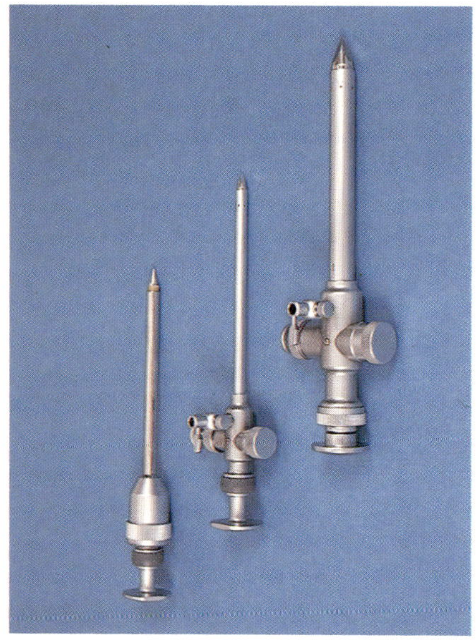

Fig. 3.8

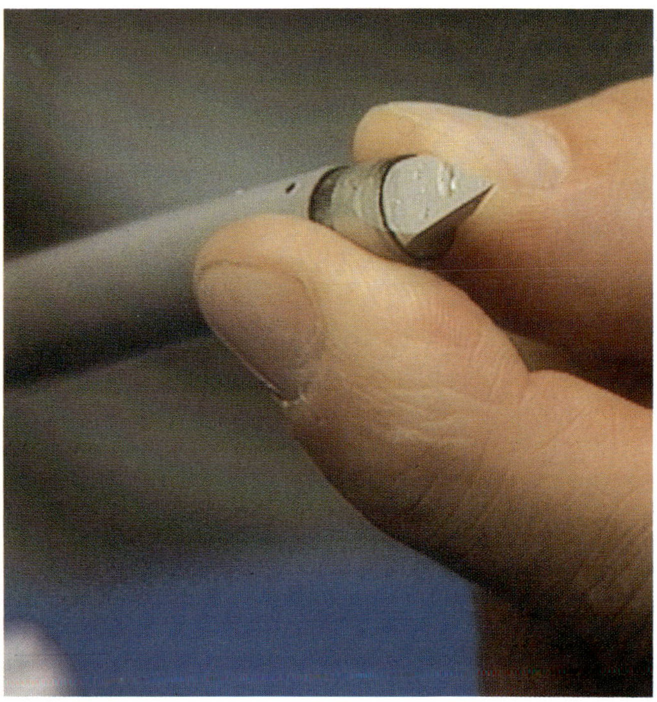

Fig. 3.9

Fig. 3.7 Two disposable laparoscopic ports, each consisting of a trocar, with safety shield, and cannula.

Fig. 3.8 A nondisposable laparoscopic port, consisting of a trocar and cannula.

Fig. 3.9 The retractable safety shield at the tip of a disposable laparoscope port is held back in this view. The shield covers the sharp trocar as soon as it enters the peritoneum.

intra-abdominal pressure seems to produce less haemodynamic instability, prevent congestion of low-pressure venous capillary beds and certainly does not splint the diaphragm to any great extent.

Ports

The term 'port' has has come into use to refer to the combination of

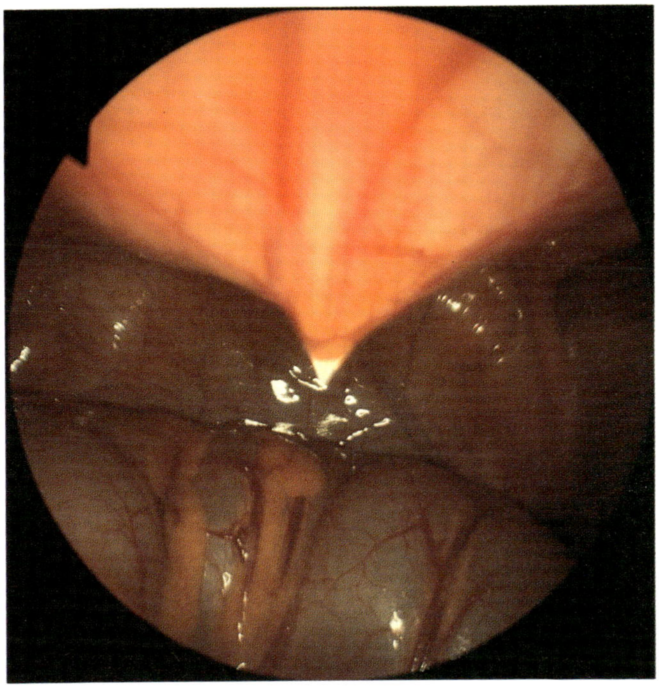

Fig. 3.10 An endoscopic view showing the sharp trocar of the disposable port penetrating the peritoneum.

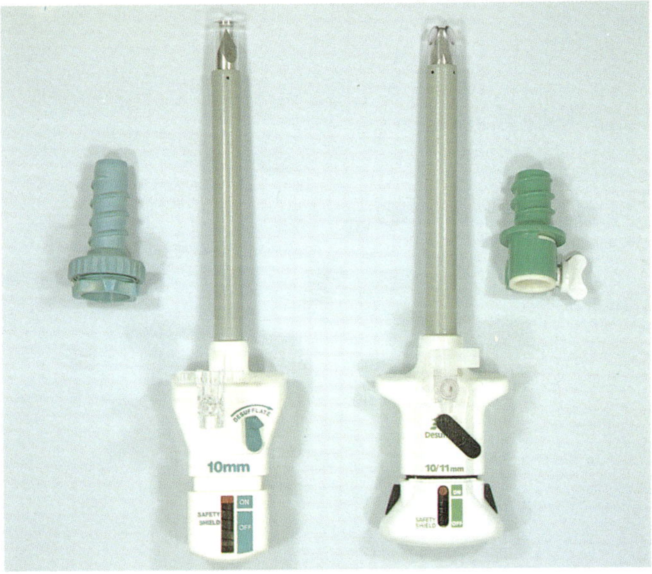

Fig. 3.11 Grips can be used to hold the laparoscopic port within the muscle fascia.

trocar and cannula. There are both nondisposable and disposable ports (Figs 3.7, 3.8). Flap valves, which are found almost exclusively in disposable ports, are superior to trumpet valves which tend to strip diathermy insulation off hand instruments. They also allow easier insertion of instruments, and the insertion of instruments single-handed.

The advantages of the flap valve, together with the incorporation of a retractable safety shield (Figs 3.9, 3.10) to cover the trocar tip once it has penetrated the peritoneum, justifies the routine use of disposable ports for the primary or telescope port at least. If finances are limited, the use of a disposable primary port and nondisposable secondary ports is a relatively inexpensive but safe compromise. The use of tissue grips on all ports to prevent inadvertant displacement is essential in all but diagnostic laparoscopic procedures (Fig. 3.11).

Probably the most important decision to be made is whether to use disposable or reusable ports and hand instruments or to compromise and to use a mixture. This has very considerable cost implications. For example, the extra cost of disposable equipment necessary to perform a laparoscopic varicocelectomy and a laparoscopic nephrectomy at 1992 prices is £417 and £917 respectively. This cost can be considerably reduced by using certain 'essential' disposables (such as the Veress needle, primary-port and insulated scissors) in conjunction with reusable equipment.

Although the overriding arbiter is often budget, other important factors are reliability, instrument performance (such as scissor or trocar sharpness) and handling, potential for cross-patient contamination and ease of cleaning. Whether choosing disposable or reusable equipment, the best advice is to spend as much money as is available and to buy only good-quality instruments.

A Hasson blunt-tipped port (Fig. 3.12) (see Chapter 4, General laparoscopic techniques) is essential when previous abdominal scars suggest adhesions. A nondisposable type is recommended, because a safety shield is not required.

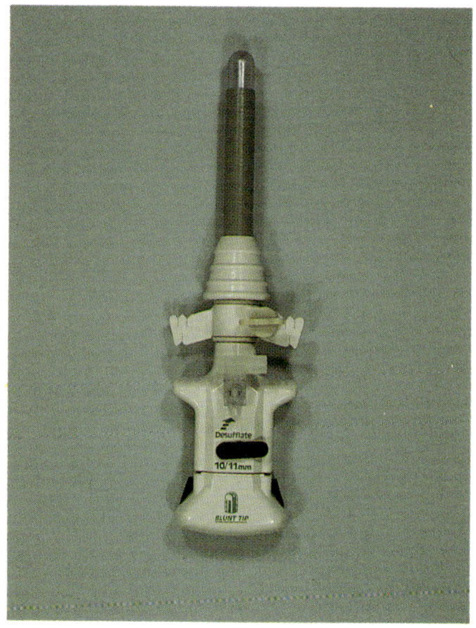

Fig. 3.12 A Hasson blunt-tipped port can be introduced by a minilaparotomy incision when abdominal scars suggest adhesions.

Manipulative instruments

The variety of manipulative instruments for laparoscopy is increasing all the time, and each new conference sees the introduction of an even greater variety. In many cases we are seeing the conversion of standard open manipulative instruments to a size and form suitable for laparoscopy. The small surface area of contact on tissues allowed for each of these instruments means that their roles are much more specific.

It is now possible to obtain a wide variety of tissue-holding forceps, retractors, dissection instruments, needle-holders and probes (Figs 3.13–3.15).

Fig. 3.13 Laparoscopic forceps: (a) soft-tissue forceps, (b) Babcock forceps.

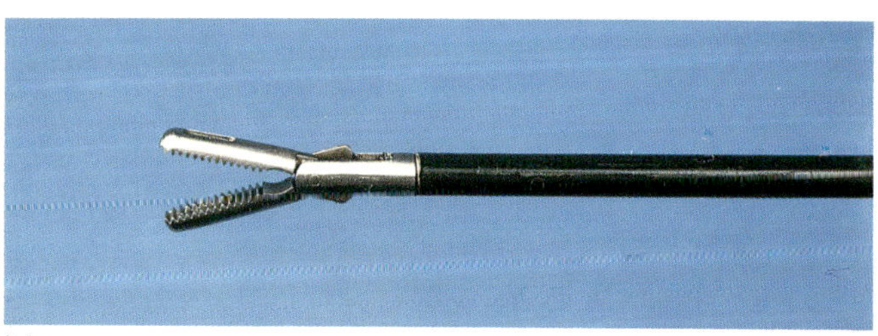

(a)

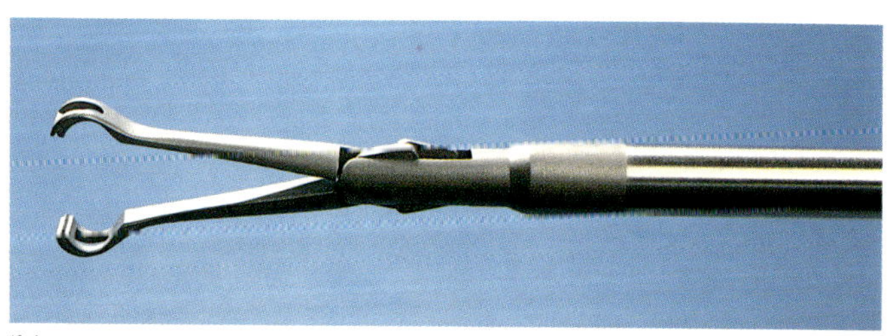

(b)

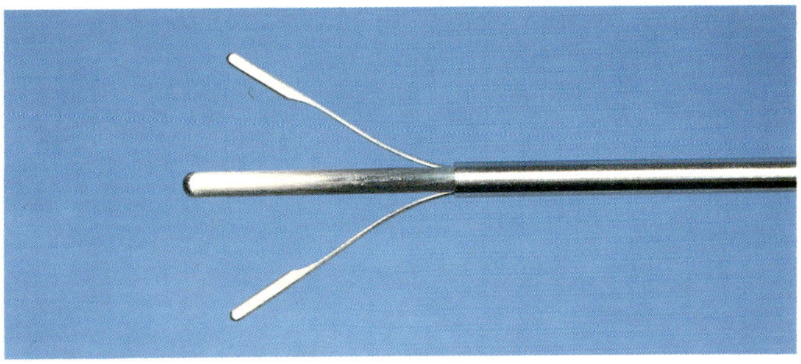

Fig. 3.14 A laparoscopic fan retractor.

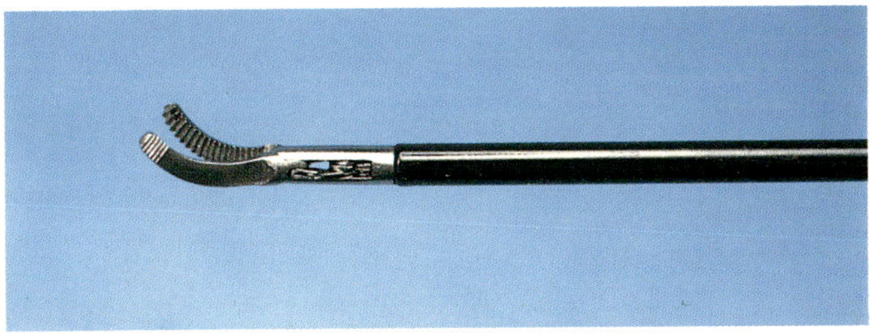

Fig. 3.15 A laparoscopic curved dissector.

One of the great difficulties in operative laparoscopy is the retraction of tissues away from the site of operation. One does not have the benefits of the size 8 assistant's hand nor a wet pack under a ring retractor. It is the introduction of various ingenious retraction devices that is now allowing us to carry out much more complex laparoscopic surgery in urology.

We have carried out an objective assessment of various laparoscopic manipulation instruments.

The handle-closure force needed to produce a 1 kg force at the jaws of five instruments of varying design with conventional handles (Fig. 3.16) was measured. This was achieved using two opposed spring balances applied to the handle blades and a calibrated force transducer between the instrument's jaws. The force needed to open the jaws of two spring-handled instruments was also measured by applying a

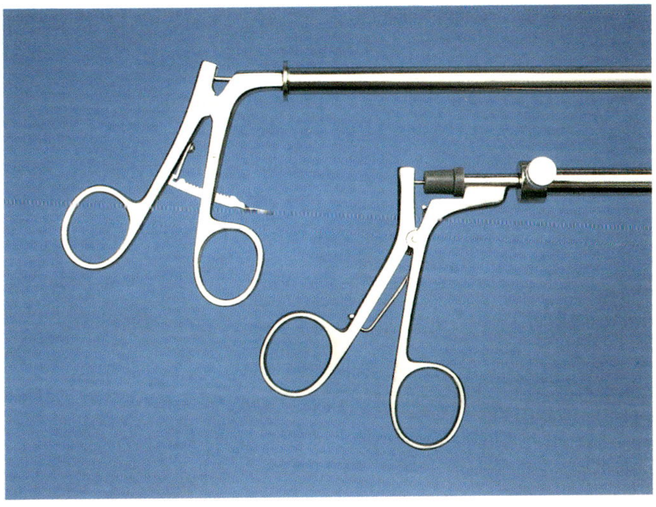

Fig. 3.16 Two conventional designs for instrument handles: ratchet-adjusted (top) and spring-handled (bottom).

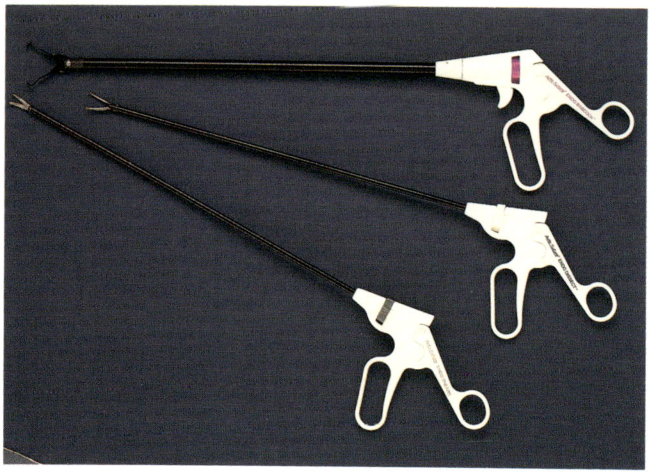

Fig. 3.17 Several optional disposable endoscopic instruments are available. The most superior of these are the endoshears. Disposable laparoscopic endoshears are sharp and insulated for monopolar diathermy application. To prevent unnecessary blunting of the blades, diathermy should only be applied through closed shears.

force to the spring while the instrument was resting on electronic scales. Additionally, we measured the closure force needed to cut a single piece of paper (80 gsm) with two scissors (one fine-curved and one heavy-hooked) using a spring balance. Each experiment was repeated three times.

There was no significant difference in mechanical advantage (force generated at the jaws or force applied to the handles) amongst the conventionally-handled instruments. Instruments with a variety of handle designs, incorporating different ratchet systems were examined; including conventional scissor-pattern handle (for use with forearm in neutral or supinated positions); spring handle; pistol grip and pen grip.

The handle design *per se* was felt to be unimportant functionally but the design of the ratchet significantly influenced the ease of operation, particularly when held in the nondominant hand. Although they required the greatest force to open the jaws, spring-handled instruments were the easiest to release. The horizontal ratchet was the most difficult to release with the vertical ratchet falling between the two.

Extra-short instruments were often found to be too short unless the ports were sited immediately over the operation site, which in turn often made for a more difficult dissection. The use of extra-long instruments produced an exaggerated shake artefact and resulted in clumsier tissue manipulation.

As there is no significant difference in mechanical advantage amongst the conventionally handled instruments, the final choice depends very much on the feel of the instrument, the features offered (especially the facility for diathermy), user-friendliness and budget. Our preference for the dominant hand is for instruments which are insulated and have rotatable shafts. Operating a ratchet with the non-dominant hand is awkward and slow and we recommend the use of spring-handled grasping forceps for this task.

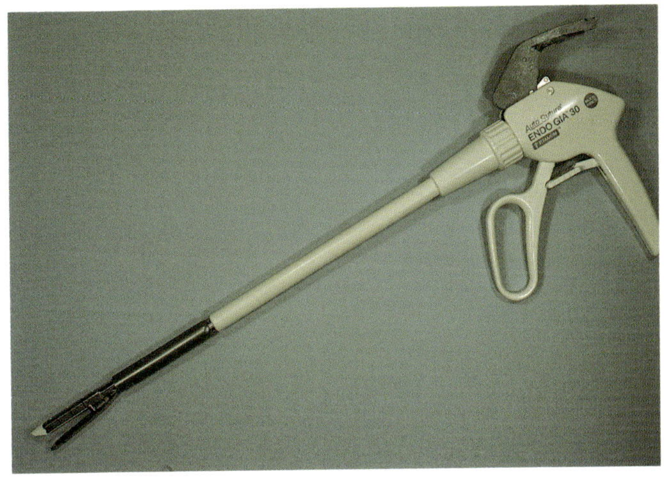

Fig. 3.18 The Endo GIA* 30 stapler and incisor is one of several options available for haemostasis. It provides secure haemostasis for blood vessels greater than 5 mm in diameter.

The use of disposable diathermy scissors (Fig. 3.17) ensures predictable, efficient and precise cutting and aids fast and accurate dissection, and this is probably the only essential disposable manipulative instrument.

Sutures

Semm pioneered the technique of laparoscopic suturing. He employed this for the re-anastomosis of a Fallopian tube, using a 2/0 gauge catgut on a short 1 cm straight needle. There are now many more sutures available for use with laparoscopic needle-holders.

In particular, there is a selection of sutures available from Ethicon which utilize a quarter-curved needle called the Ski needle. This has the advantage that it can be introduced through a 5 mm laparoscopic port but also is curved enough to be an aid to anastomotic suturing. All types of suture material have been made available by Ethicon with this round-bodied needle.

Laparoscopic suturing can be quite time-consuming and there are many instances, particularly with regard to small-bowel anastomoses, when the Endo GIA 30 stapler (Fig. 3.18) is much faster and just as safe. This instrument from AutoSuture is available in a 3 cm form, thus requiring at least two applications to provide a suitable anastomotic lumen; a 6 cm cartridge is due to be introduced in the near future. Similar staplers will soon be available from Ethicon. At the present time, a small-bowel re-anastomosis during the formation of an ileal conduit requires at least 4 fires of the Endo GIA 30 stapler.

Haemostatic devices

Monopolar diathermy current used from either the dissecting scissors

*A trademark of the United States Surgical Corporation (AutoSuture).

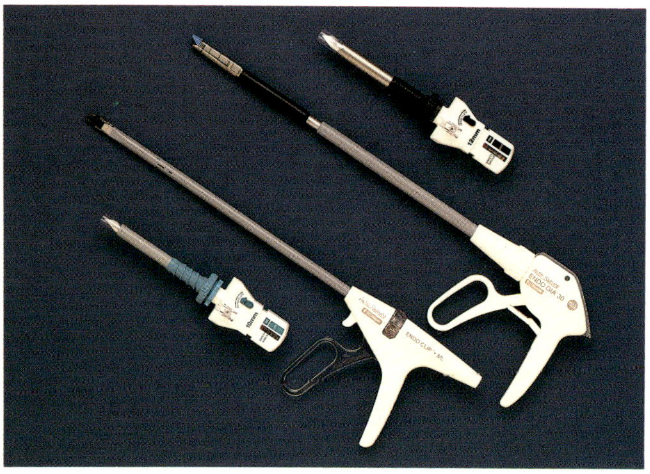

Fig. 3.19 A disposable Endoclip Applier. To achieve secure haemostasis, it is important to visualize the opposing clip ends across a well-dissected vessel .

or separate laparoscopic forceps is a method commonly employed for vessels up to 2mm in diameter. Beyond this, and certainly for arterial haemostasis, one requires mechanical clipping devices. Three sorts are available and these have been evaluated in our department by Eden and Popert.

The recent enthusiasm for laparoscopic surgery has resulted in the development and refinement of a variety of mechanical haemostatic devices. To date, there are no guidelines for the use of these devices. Eden's and Popert's study establishes such guidelines and has considerable cost implications.

A series of bursting pressure-vessel diameter curves were constructed using mesenteric arteries of two-year-old sheep and three commercially available occlusive devices. The haemostatic devices assessed were:

1 Medium-large Endoclip Applier (AutoSuture) (Fig. 3.19)
2 Lockable PDS AP400 clip (Ethicon)
3 Endo GIA 30 stapler (AutoSuture)

The bursting pressure was measured for each device on arteries with external diameters of 3mm, 5mm, 7mm and 9mm. Each experiment was conducted using static and pulsatile flow and was repeated at least three times.

All three devices could be applied securely up to a vessel diameter of 5mm, withstanding a pressure of 500cmH_2O. Beyond this diameter, the clip did not totally occlude the vessel lumen.

The maximum diameter vessel which could be accommodated in the jaws of the PDS clip was 7mm. The vessel withstood a pressure of 500cmH_2O. The Endo GIA 30 stapler occluded vessels of all sizes and also withstood a pressure of 500cmH_2O. The clips can be applied safely to vessels up to 5mm in diameter and they are provided in a multifire cartridge.

Lockable PDS AP400 clips should be used for larger vessels up to 7mm in diameter, but have the practical disadvantage of having to be loaded singly. The use of the Endo GIA 30 stapler should be reserved for vessels greater than 7mm in diameter, such as renal artery and vein.

Water-jet dissectors

Semm was the first to introduce a combined instrument for saline irrigation and aspiration. This instrument is very helpful for removing small amounts of blood. However, it is necessary always to remember that during aspiration, the tip of the probe must be kept under the fluid level or you will witness a rapid decompression of the pneumoperitoneum.

Many companies have increased the pressure of irrigation and termed the new inspiration a dissector. The concept is that the probe is then placed in the subperitoneal tissues and the reflux of saline dissects away the fat leaving the vessels and other structures free.

These modifications have not always been helpful, because the resultant tissues can be much more difficult to manipulate. Without doubt we will see such instruments refined in the near future, for they do hold great promise.

Lasers and diathermy

There was a great debate during the advent of the laparoscopic cholecystectomy as to whether laser or diathermy dissection was more efficient and safer. This was an argument fuelled by several laser companies who saw that their sales had been dwindling and expected a new market to open up to them, especially if they donated a laser to key clinicians.

The Nd:YAG laser combined with a sapphire tip has never been anything other than an expensive form of monopolar diathermy and both can be used for dissection and coagulation of vessels up to 1mm in diameter without any coaptation. Using either of these energy forms for dissection causes unnecessary local increases in heat and misting of the telescope, and endoscopic scissors with diathermy, directed through the scissors, are greatly to be preferred when small vessels are visually encountered. This enables a much cleaner form of dissection. It is important to keep the scissors closed when using diathermy to prevent blunting when the current takes the route of least resistance across the sharp blade.

Retrieval devices

These are in essence simple impermeable bags (Fig. 3.21) which are used to collect organs and tissue within the abdomen and bring them safely onto the abdominal wall via one of the ports (Fig. 3.22). They

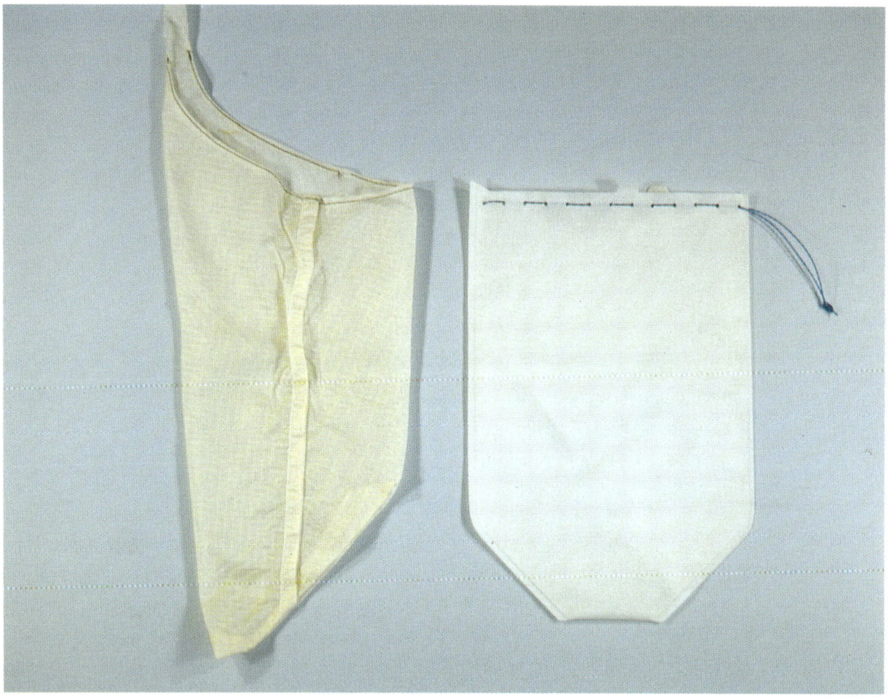

Fig. 3.20 Two designs of kidney retrieval bag. The bags are impermeable to cellular fluid and are made of rip-proof nylon.

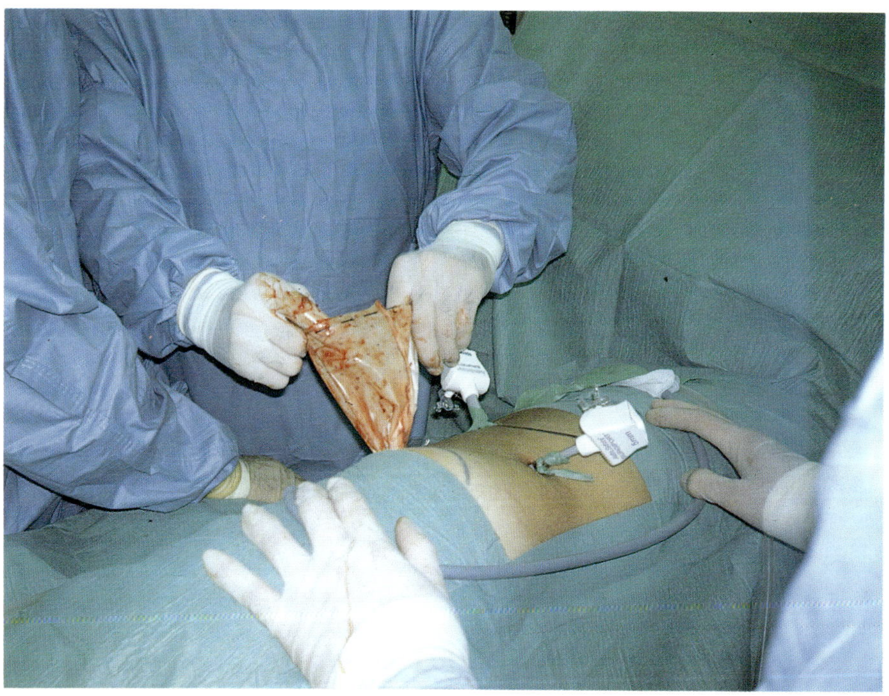

Fig. 3.21 The neck of the retrieval bag has been brought out on to the abdominal wall during a nephrectomy, prior to morcellation within the bag.

were first introduced for infected or 'hot' gall bladders but are now used for the removal of bowel tumours and end organs such as the ovary, kidney and spleen.

They are much more than just a bag in that they must be of such a design that can be easily introduced through a port and be strong enough to withstand the morcellation that is required when tissue is

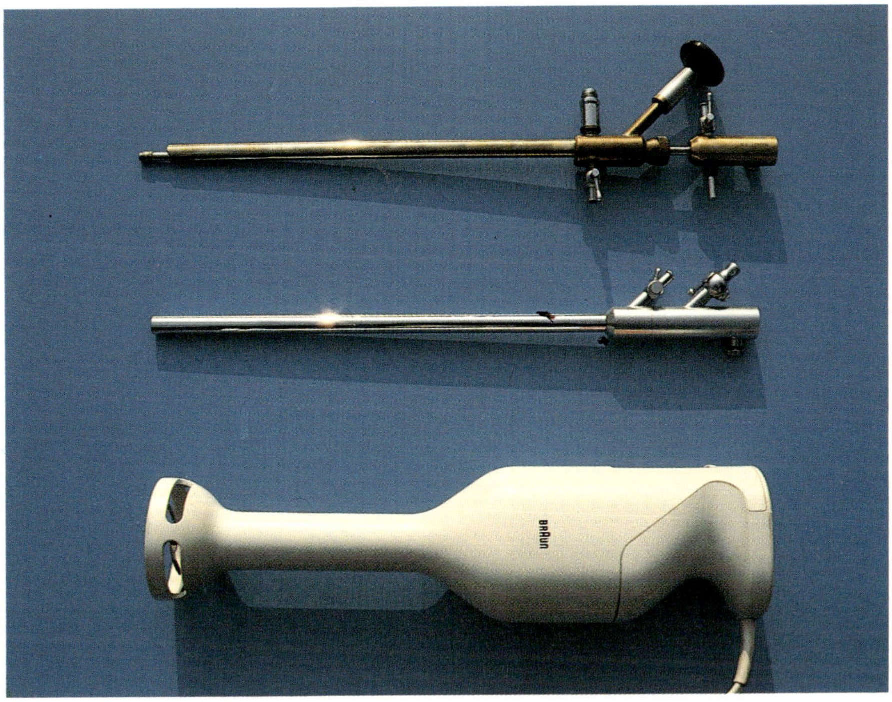

Fig. 3.22 The endoscopic liquidizer and surgical aspirator (middle). It has been used to morcellate nephrectomy specimens within the retrieval bag but, like many of its counterparts, is often obstructed by fibrous tissue components. The principle, based on a kitchen blender (bottom), has also been used for a 5 mm endoscopic device for the prostate (top).

too bulky to bring out directly through the abdominal wall. Impermeability to all cells is also essential.

Once the neck of the retrieval bag has been brought out to the surface, then any further dissection or morcellation becomes extracorporeal and there is no danger of seeding possible tumour cells back into the peritoneum.

Morcellating devices

Morcellating devices are required when the tissue bulk is greater than the diameter of the port. There are a variety of crude devices available at the moment, and we are certain to see a great refinement of these in the near future. At present, the main problem is the morcellation and removal of fibrous connective tissue, which causes the instrument to malfunction. At present, there is not very much difference between inserting a pair of blunt-nosed Mayo scissors and fragmenting the tissue and the electrical devices which either liquidize or morcellate the tissue (Fig. 3.22).

One of the disadvantages of removing tissue in a liquidized or morcellated state is that accurate staging of a possible tumour by the histopathologist is very difficult, if not sometimes impossible. This means that preoperative staging must be as thorough as possible and in the case of renal tumours, a CT scan is essential in every case when previously one might have operated solely with an IVU and ultrasound. However, the type of tissue and possible tumour can easily be identified even with liquidized samples.

References

KeyMed (1992) Optical tests for comparison of laparoscopes/video systems. KeyMed (Medical and Industrial Equipment) Ltd.

O'Boyle P. (1990) Videoendoscopy. The remote operating technique. *British Journal of Urology*, **65**, 557–9.

4: General Laparoscopic Techniques

M.J. COPTCOAT AND A.D. JOYCE

Introduction

The peritoneum is the largest and most complex serous membrane in the body. The part lining the abdominal wall (parietes) is called the parietal peritoneum, whilst that lining the viscera is the visceral peritoneum. The parietal and visceral layers are in actual contact and are lubricated by a small quantity of serous fluid which allows them to glide over each other. The insufflating gas is injected into the potential space between the two layers, called the peritoneal cavity.

The parietal peritoneum is only loosely applied to the abdominal wall anteriorly, where it derives its blood supply and innervation. Since these nerves carry sensory information in A delta somatic fibres to the dorsal columns of the spinal cord, injury or irritation of the parietal peritoneum produces acute or 'sharp' pain. It can be abolished with local anaesthesia for insertion of trocars but although this is adequate for diagnostic laparoscopy, muscle paralysis is essential for free manipulation of multiple instruments which in turn necessitates a general anaesthetic with ventilation. Assisted ventilation is also useful in artificially reversing the acidosis that can occur from prolonged carbon dioxide absorption. Thus you have the apparent anomaly of a day-case minimally invasive procedure that requires paralysis and assisted ventilation.

On the other hand, the visceral peritoneum is very closely applied to the viscera it invests and from which it receives its blood supply and innervation. These nerves carry sensory information in C fibres of the sympathetic nervous system and do not cause pain in response to direct injury such as burning or clipping but rather to stretching and distension which is minimal during laparoscopic procedures.

Laparoscopic inspection of the peritoneal cavity requires identification and opening up of the potential space between the visceral and parietal peritoneal layers. The space can be difficult to find, especially in the obese and in patients who have undergone previous intra-abdominal surgery with subsequent adhesion formation. Early pioneers placed their first port through a minilaparotomy, but with the advent of the safe Veress needle, a simple and safe technique can be quickly mastered for the majority of patients and a minilaparotomy reserved for those with adhesions.

Once the needle is in the correct compartment, flow of gas must be sufficient to maintain an adequate space for inspection and surgery. Following the introduction of the gas into the peritoneal cavity, the intracavity pressure rises to a level which depends on the volume of gas and the compliance of the cavity. Lower pressures are necessary to achieve good visualization when the abdominal wall is completely relaxed and the passively distended abdomen forms a marquee in which the surgery is performed with an audience. Pressures of 10 cmH_2O are usually deemed adequate. Higher pressures may exceed capillary pressure and prevent absorption of gas into the portal and systemic circulation but locally produce unwanted congestion and difficult haemostasis.

Operating theatre layout

Operative laparoscopy is high technology, and whilst the urologist should be familiar with all of his or her equipment, there is no doubt that the success of complicated laparoscopic procedures depends on the whole team. Nursing staff and technicians may need to receive specialized training in the care and maintenance of new equipment. Simple advice, such as avoiding pointed towel clips when stabilizing camera and light leads, is vital to prevent damage but is not usually part of the standard operating nurse training.

The position of the patient, operator and assistant has been described for each separate technique in this book. The monitors should always be placed directly opposite the operator and assistant. A slave monitor for the assistant is ergonomically much more satisfactory. Racked systems which include light source, insufflator, camera unit and video recorder occupy less space but it is important always to keep the diathermy machine as far away from the imaging system as possible to reduce diathermy interference. The ideal position for the scrub nurse will vary for each surgeon especially if this nurse is also acting as an assistant. The scrub nurse must also have easy access to a laparotomy set, which must always be available. It will seldom be used, but when it is required, it will probably be for an emergency.

Despite all of these extra lessons that need to be learned by both urologists and nurses alike, these are exciting times to be involved in operative laparoscopy. The principles have become established and the opportunity is there for all to contribute in refining our techniques and sharing universally in a surgical subspecialty that is rewarding to participate in, fun to watch and is definitely the way ahead.

Formation of a pneumoperitoneum

The common starting point for all laparoscopic procedures is the formation of a pneumoperitoneum. The initial puncturing needle through which gas is insufflated has traditionally been called a Veress

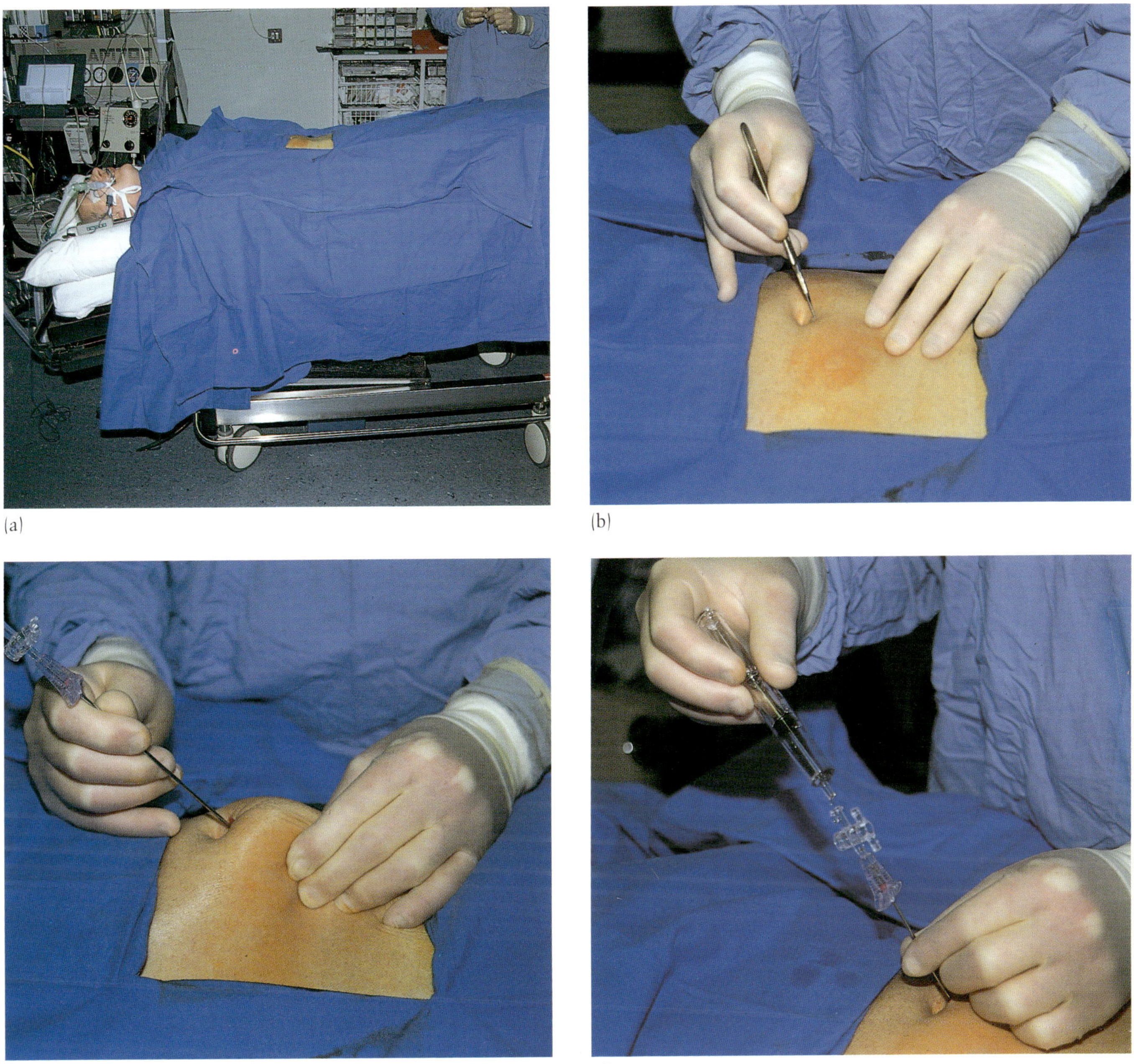

(a) (b) (c) (d)

Fig. 4.1 Preparations for creating a pneumoperitoneum for pelvic laparoscopy. (a) The patient is prepared in a 25% head-down position. (b) A hemicircular incision is made below the umbilicus. (c) The Veress needle is inserted at 45° into the pelvis, whilst the abdomen wall is lifted. (d) The needle position is checked with the drop test (see main text).

needle. This is also available as a disposable needle with the same safety mechanism as the trocars and cannulae. The needle is held as a dart and pushed into the abdominal space, helped by the pulling up of a fold of the abdomen (Fig. 4.1c). There are three quick tests that strongly suggest that the needle has been satisfactorily positioned. First, aspirate. Secondly, infuse 3–5 ml of saline. There should be no resistance. Finally, witness a drop of saline receding down the needle because of the relative vacuum created by lifting up the abdominal wall (Fig. 4.1d). These tests have a small false negative rate and it is interesting that our gynaecological colleagues rarely use them. The

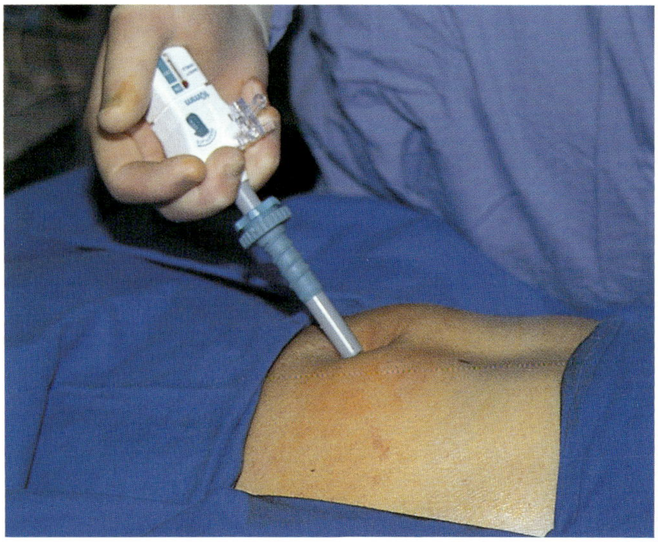

(a)

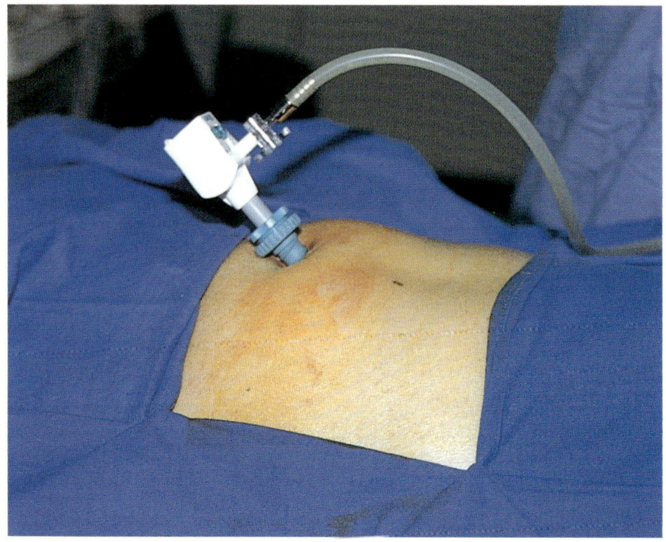

(b)

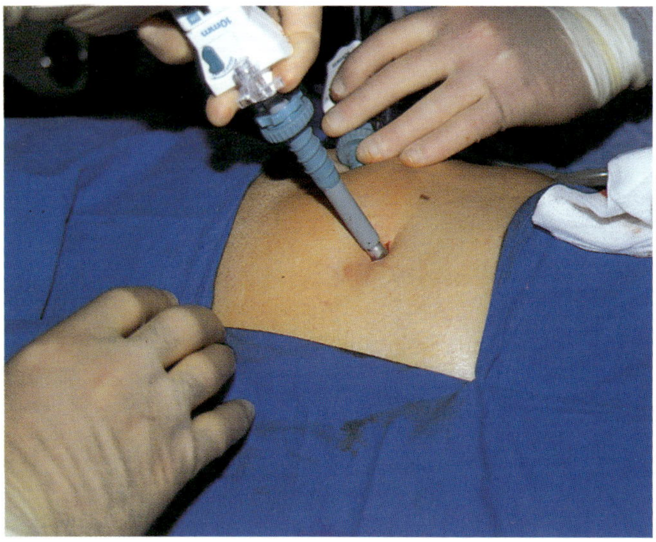

(c)

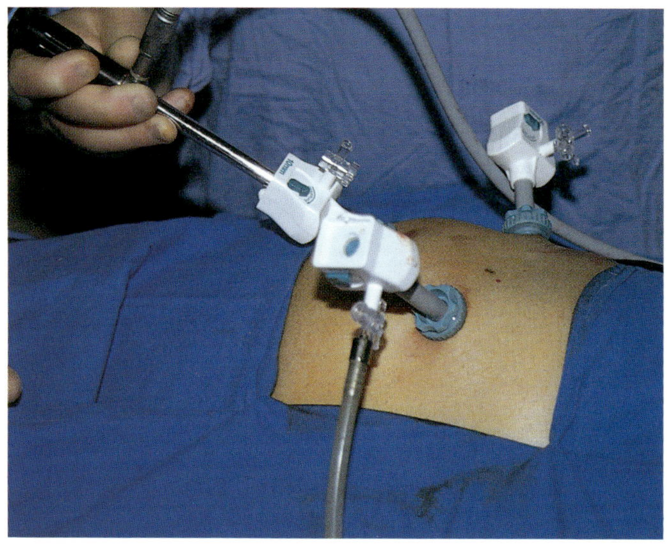

(d)

Fig. 4.2 Placement the telescope port and secondary ports. (a) A 10mm disposable port is inserted below the umbilicus for the telescope. (b) Carbon dioxide is initially transferred to the telescope port. (c) Secondary ports are inserted. (d) Carbon dioxide is connected to a secondary port to prevent cooling of the telescope.

needle is then connected to a gas insufflator. Modern insufflators not only provide varying flow rates and a measure of the volume and pressure infused but can also be set to an automatic mode which is invaluable during long procedures. If the initial infusion pressure is above 10mm of mercury then one must suspect that the Veress needle is not lying free within the abdomen or is trapped in omentum or behind bowel. This can usually be corrected by simple repositioning of the tip. Subsequent pressures again should not exceed 10mm of mercury because it is felt that this would severely impede the venous return through intra-abdominal organs over a period of several hours and increase the splinting effect on the diaphragm. However, this is very much a theoretical concept, and work still needs to be done concerning the possible hazards of very long laparoscopic procedures. Up until now, we have, perhaps naively, felt that the anaesthetic risks of

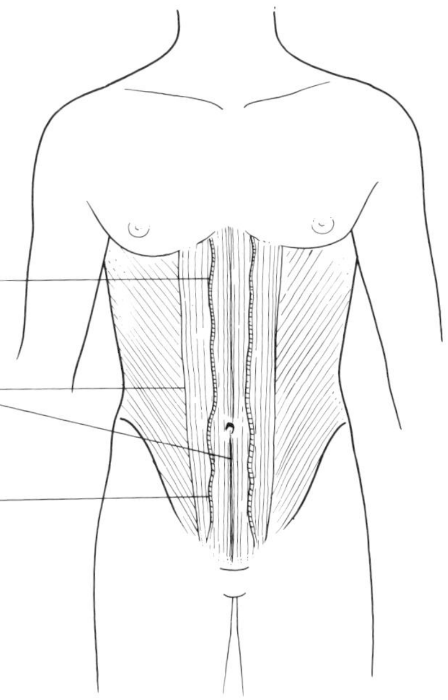

Fig. 4.3 The inferior epigastric artery coursing along the rectus sheath, anastomosing with the superior epigastric artery, is the source of frustrating complications of secondary port placement. The ideal port sites are in the midline or at the edge of the rectus sheath in the semilunar line.

a long laparoscopic nephrectomy were similar to the transatlantic crossing by a jumbo jet where the only dangers are concerned with the very beginning and end of the procedure.

Port placement

A 10 or 12mm trocar and cannula is then inserted into the abdomen for initial laparoscopic viewing (Fig. 4.2a). This is traditionally done through a small skin incision on the periphery of the umbilicus. This site has mainly been used for its cosmetic advantages and we are now finding that there are many instances when the camera should be placed elsewhere.

One golden rule to follow is that the viewing laparoscope, with or without its associated camera, should be inserted away from the site of operation. This provides the potential for both close-up and distant wide-angle views once several instruments are in the operative field. The sites of the midline and semilunar lines are chosen because of the absence of muscle at these potential points of entry and both are guaranteed to miss the superficial epigastric vessels which run up through the rectus muscles (Fig. 4.3). Subsequent ports should always be sited after internal illumination with the house lights off. This shows that one is clear of abdominal wall vessels. A transverse skin incision is made which will form a snug fit around the cannula and grip. The ports should be inserted under direct endoscopic vision and removal of ports should also be visualized in case a vessel had been perforated that will haemorrhage postoperatively without the tamponading effect of the cannula. Grips that hold the port firmly in the muscle fascia are preferred because one can safely withdraw all but

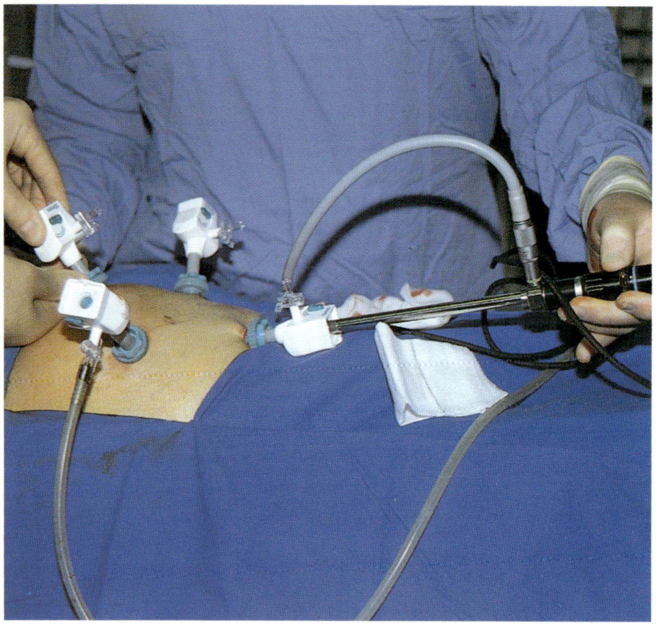

Fig. 4.4 The position of the telescope port grip is checked by looking retrogradely from a secondary port.

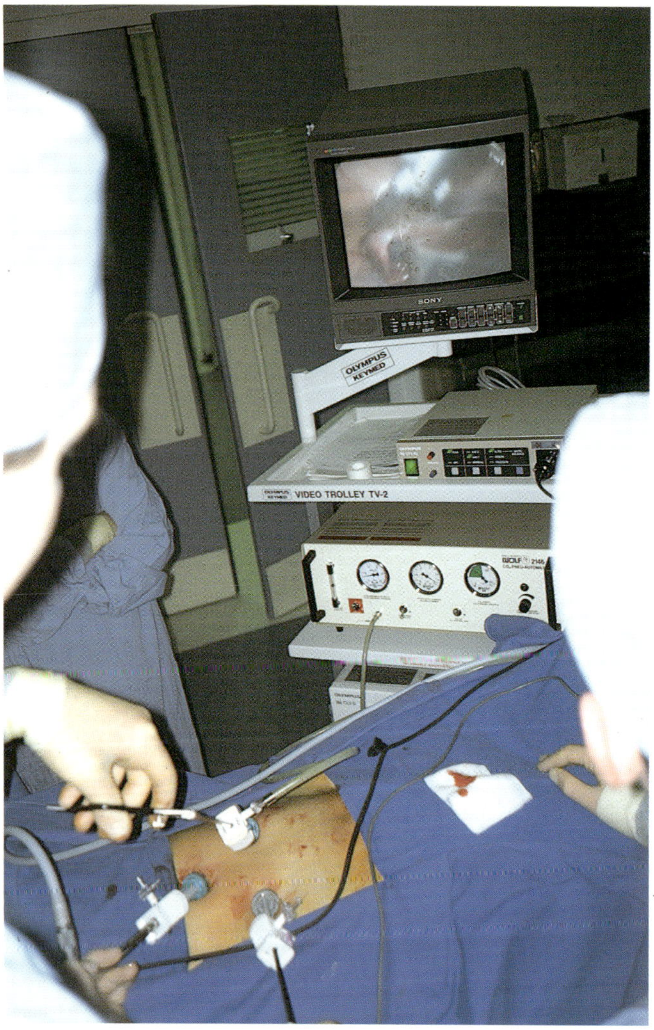

Fig. 4.5 With the pneumoperitoneum achieved, and all the ports in place, operative video laparoscopy can begin.

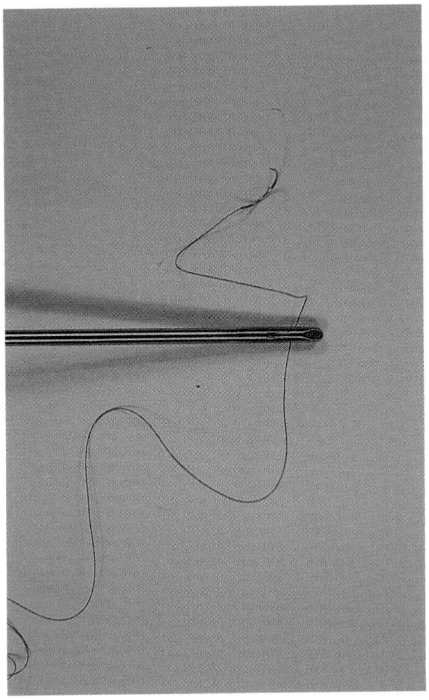

Fig. 4.6 The laparoscopic suture should be grasped 3–4 cm proximal to the needle. Then even a curved needle can be pulled through a port if the valve is momentarily depressed.

1 cm of the port from the abdomen. This produces a greater range for forceps to open and allows the telescope to provide a very wide field of view when required.

Laparoscopic suturing techniques

Laparoscopic suturing is a difficult technique, and at the present time there is little need for it in urological laparoscopy. However, unexpected situations may be encountered such as an omental tear or bowel perforation during a difficult trocar insertion. Having been presented with a patient requiring a nephrectomy who had undergone three previous major abdominal operations, Coptcoat found the pneumoperitoneum to be straightforward but insertion of the first trocar very difficult. Adhesions held the transverse colon close to the abdominal wall and a perforation was made with this trocar. This was recognized during initial inspection when he found that he was viewing the inside of the large bowel rather than the peritoneal cavity. Insertion of two ports adjacent to this area allowed him to inspect the iatrogenic bowel perforation. The perforation could be oversewn with two layers of interrupted sutures using an intracorporeal technique. The transperitoneal laparoscopic nephrectomy could then go ahead as planned. Such a complication and its remedy using suturing techniques is unusual but the example provides evidence of the capabilities of such suturing techniques.

What we will undoubtedly see is an expansion of urological laparoscopy in which suture anastomoses will be the first choice until stapling anastomotic techniques are refined both in terms of instrumentation and the application of absorbable staples. At the present time, a laparoscopic pyeloplasty is best done with a continuous intracorporeal laparoscopic suture.

Generally speaking, special laparoscopic needles and sutures are not required. Most straight needles and some curved needles can easily be introduced through 10 mm ports. The suture material should be grasped with a pair of forceps approximately 3–4 cm proximal to the needle itself and the needle then dragged through the port. The flap valve, if present, should be depressed momentarily during this manoeuvre (Fig. 4.6).

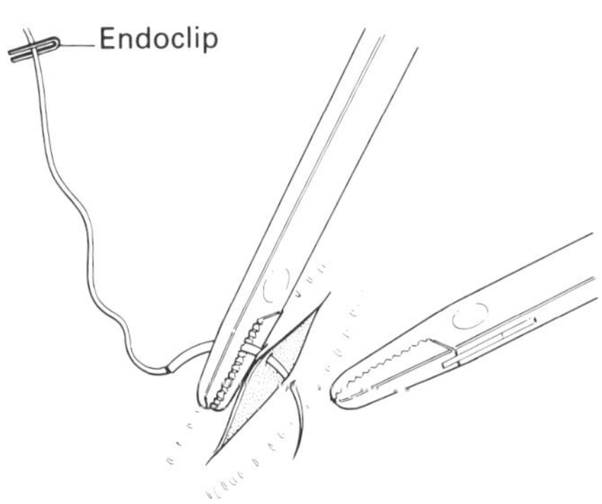

Fig. 4.7 A quick technique to start a continuous suture is to place a clip at the opposite end of the suture material to the needle. This technique can also be used to complete a continuous suture. The clip is less likely to slide off from braided sutures.

Continuous suture

The suture line is cut to the desired length. Excess suture material is difficult to handle intracorporeally. The traditional method of tying a knot at the beginning and end of the continuous suture can be reproduced within the abdomen but is tedious and time-consuming. A far quicker technique is to place a clip at the opposite end of the suture material to the needle; this is firmly tightened (Fig. 4.7). A continuous

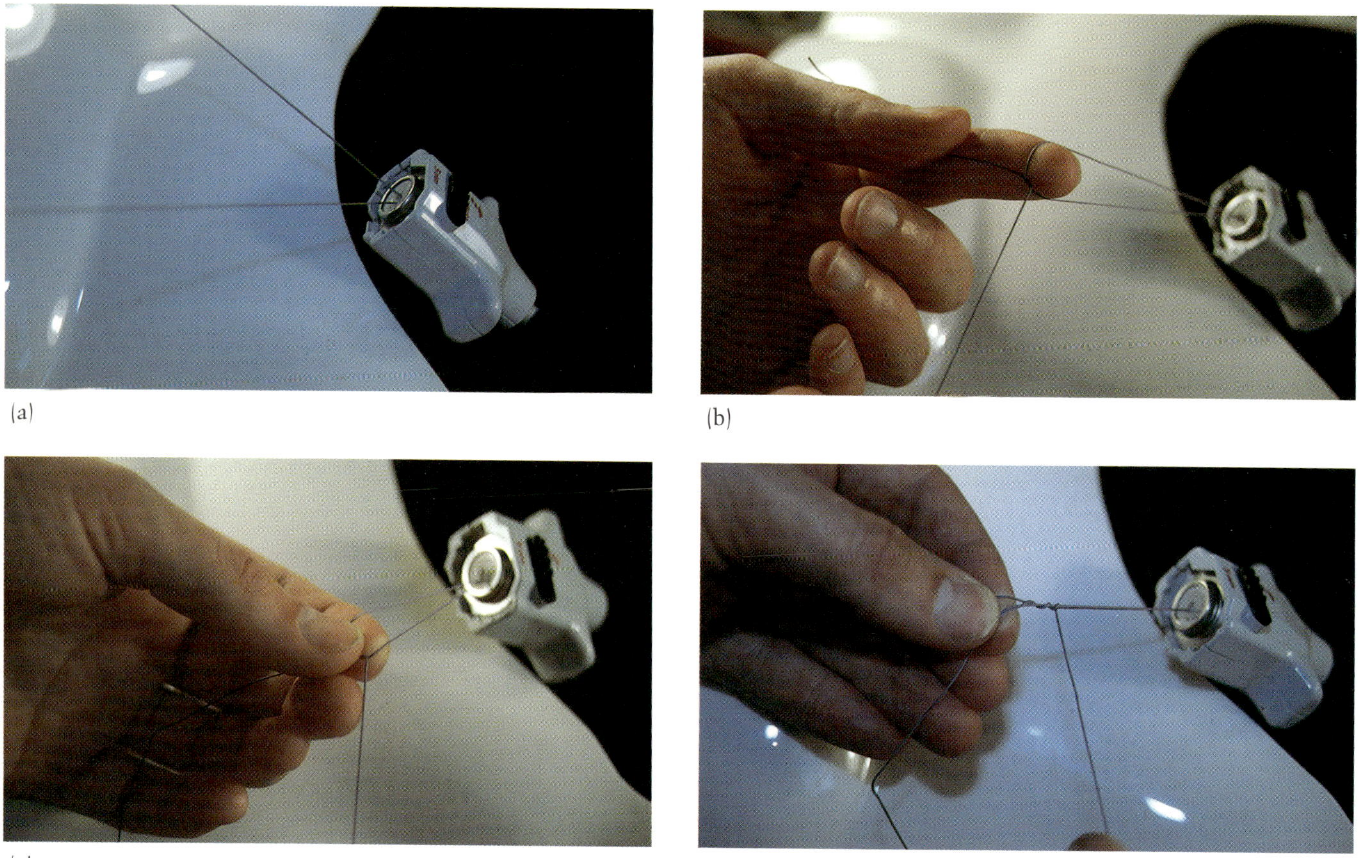

(a) (b) (c) (d)

Fig. 4.8 The extracorporeal knot technique. (a) The two ends are withdrawn through the port. (b) A single throw knot is made. (c) The throw knot is held with thumb and second finger. (d) Three revolutions are made around both strands. (e) This knot is recommended when using monofilament suture materials. (f) The lust is pushed down with a knot tier. (g) The suture is then finished and cut.

suture is made using an endoscopic needle-holder and a grasper. The function of the grasping forceps is to present the needle in the right position in relation to the needle-holder, to grasp the needle when it is passed through the tissue and to control the tension on the suture as it is drawn through the tissue. It also helps to depress the tissue at the anticipated needle exit point should the needle tip be too difficult to see. This provides a better exposure of the needle. A wider field panoramic view is more desirable for suturing because of the relatively wide arc of movements that the instruments follow. When the continuous suture is finished, it is fastened off with a clip and cut. This technique allows for a suture line of only a few centimetres thus making the manipulation easier.

Interrupted suture

Numerous techniques of knot-tying have been described, including intracorporeal and extracorporeal procedures.

The intracorporeal technique requires intensive training and practice but has few indications in urological laparoscopy. It is possible to tie almost all of the sutures outside of the abdomen. The needle is introduced into the abdomen. The opposite end can be secured outside with small forceps to avoid its accidentally sliding into the

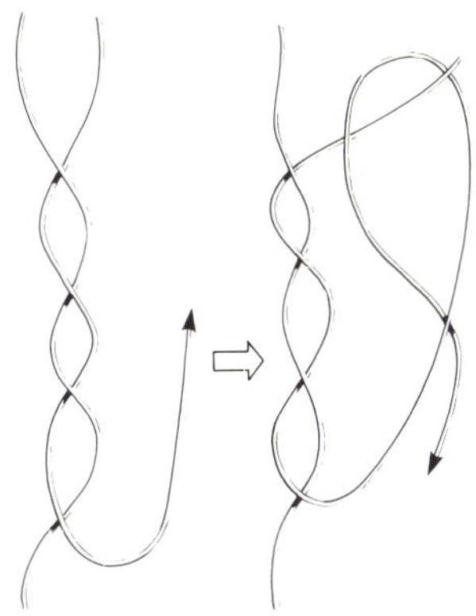

(e)

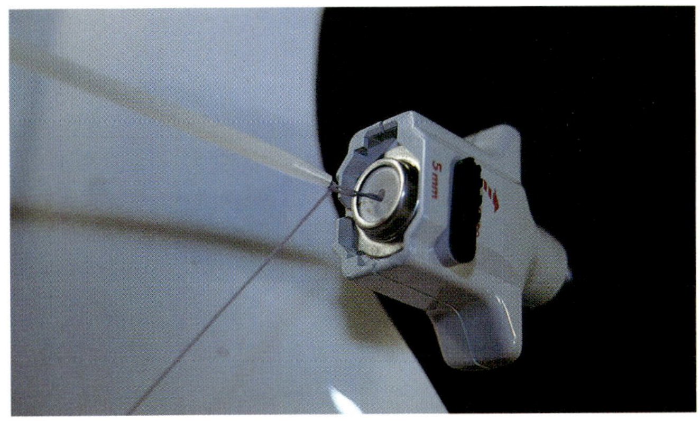

(f)

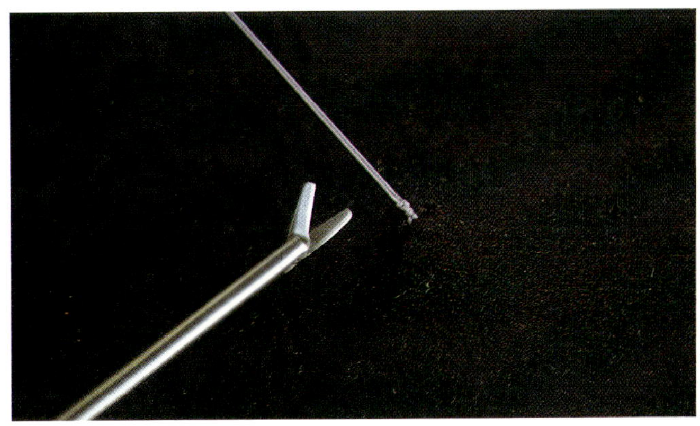

(g)

Fig. 4.8 *Contd*

operative field. The needle is passed through the tissue as previously described and then withdrawn through that same port. A single throw knot is made with the two suture ends. This knot is held with the thumb and second finger. With the free end of the suture, three revolutions are made around both suture strands. The tail of the suture is inserted through the first loop and then though the loop that was formed below the initial single throw knot. This is a fisherman's knot (Fig. 4.8). The tail is pulled up and cut. By simply pulling the end of the thread, the knot slides down by itself. It is then pushed with a knot tier or atraumatic forceps and secured. Finally, the suture is cut off 3mm from the knot.

Intracorporeal knot-tying is merely a reproduction of those techniques we use at open surgery. The movements are more difficult when restricted to laparoscopic instruments and their angle of entry, but with practice and, in particular, with shorter lengths of suture material, such intracorporeal suturing can be mastered (Fig. 4.9).

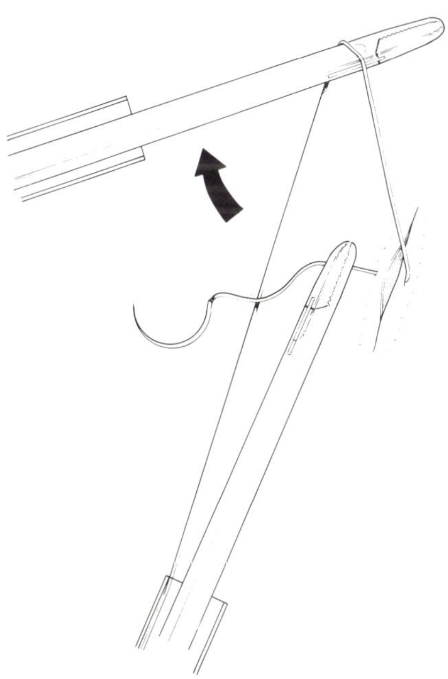

Fig. 4.9 Intracorporeal knot-tying is time-consuming, but the point of manipulation is close to the point tissue approximation, and so tears are less likely.

Wound closures

The use of larger ports (e.g. 10, 12 and 16mm) has made the possibility of a postoperative wound hernia more likely. In these instances, the wound should be closed at the end of the operation by placing a

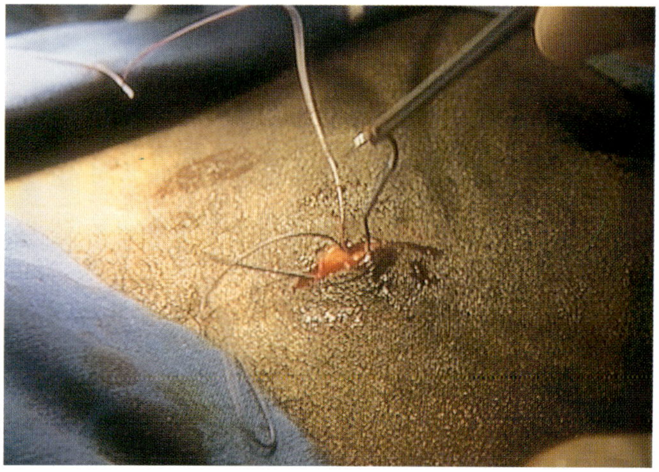

Fig. 4.10 Port wounds of 10mm or more should receive a fascial suture to prevent wound-herniation.

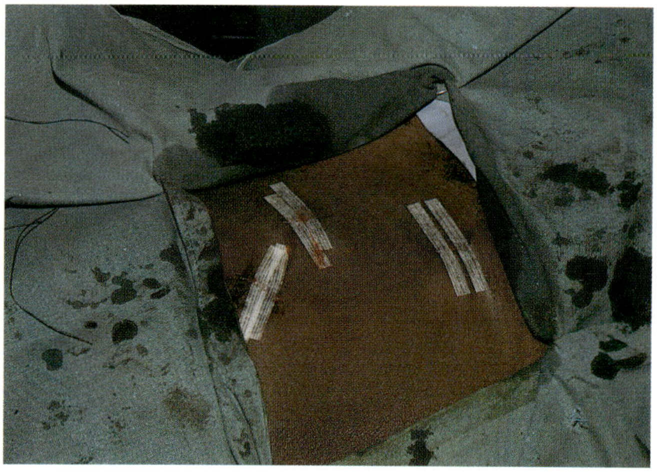

Fig. 4.11 Skin wounds can be closed with a subcuticular suture, or as in this case, with steristrips. The cosmetic result is excellent.

suture across the fascia (Fig. 4.10). If there is any difficulty in picking up the fascia externally, a large hand needle can be passed through with endoscopic guidance from below. The skin can then be closed separately either with a subcuticular suture or a steristrip (Fig. 4.11). Dexon seems to produce a slight hypertrophy of the scar which can mar the external appearance of a successful minimally invasive procedure. Something nonabsorbable is to be preferred.

5: Anaesthesia for Laparoscopy

D. GREEN AND A. MITCHELL

Introduction

Following the introduction of gynaecological laparoscopy doubts were soon expressed about the difficulties and dangers inherent in a seemingly simple and relatively noninvasive technique. As a result of investigations into the effects of peritoneal insufflation of carbon dioxide during laparoscopy, Hodgson *et al.* (1970) concluded, 'Though laparoscopy offers advantages to both patients and surgeon it involves considerable alteration in respiratory and cardiovascular homeostasis and should not be regarded as yet another minor investigation.' However, it is only with the recent introduction of more prolonged techniques, such as laparoscopic nephrectomy, that the full scale of these 'alterations' has manifested itself. Both the anaesthetist and the surgeon must be aware of the pathophysiological effects of laparoscopy so that the patient can receive optimum benefit from the technique and experience minimum complications.

Anaesthetic techniques

General anaesthetic techniques for laparoscopy do not differ markedly from those used for other surgical procedures. However, in recent years the spectrum of laparoscopic techniques has widened from simple laparoscopic sterilization in gynaecology lasting a few minutes to the more complex urological procedures, such as laparoscopic nephrectomy, which may take up to seven hours. For ambulatory procedures, opioid supplementation should be minimized as this may delay recovery and increase the risk of postoperative nausea and vomiting .

Is endotracheal intubation mandatory?

A long-standing debate regarding the necessity for endotracheal intubation (ETI) during the shorter gynaecological laparoscopic procedures has continued for the last 20 years. Since the majority of these procedures are carried out in day-surgery units, reducing the incidence of sore throat from ETI or muscle pains associated with the relaxant suxamethonium is seen as a major advantage of avoiding ETI (Kenefick *et al.* 1987).

Nevertheless, during longer procedures, the combination of a head-down tilt and pneumoperitoneum could increase the risk of regurgitation of gastric contents, especially in the obese patient. In these cases, ETI is employed.

Is mechanical ventilation mandatory?

Hypoventilation in the spontaneously breathing patient is exacerbated by a head-down tilt and diaphragmatic splinting from the pneumoperitoneum. This, together with carbon dioxide absorption (if carbon dioxide is used as the insufflating gas) leads to hypercapnea. The association of ventricular dysrhythmias, hypercapnea and halothane anaesthesia thus led to a preference for mechanical ventilation to control $PaCO_2$ during gynaecological laparoscopy (Hodgson *et al.* 1970). Although newer inhalational agents, such as isoflurane, are much less likely to cause dysrhythmias in the spontaneously breathing patient undergoing laparoscopy for shorter procedures (Kenefick *et al.* 1987), longer cases make mechanical ventilation mandatory, as carbon dioxide absorption may be considerable (Blobner *et al.* 1992).

Is muscle paralysis mandatory?

Having decided to intubate and ventilate the patient, is it necessary to maintain neuromuscular blockade throughout the procedure? During complex intra-abdominal surgery such as nephrectomy, visualization depends on adequate separation of the visceral and parietal layers of the peritoneum, and this can only be achieved by complete relaxation (high compliance) of the abdominal wall musculature, if high intra-abdominal pressures are to be avoided.

In addition, avoidance of sudden patient movement (e.g. coughing) is necessary to prevent inadvertent injury. In these cases, muscle paralysis must be sustained throughout the procedure, and the effects of the neuromuscular blocker must be monitored with a peripheral nerve stimulator.

Is nitrous oxide contraindicated?

Concerns have been expressed over the use of nitrous oxide during prolonged laparoscopic surgery because of its puted ability to cause bowel distension which might hinder surgical access (Eger & Saidman 1965, Marco *et al.* 1990) and a puted increased risk of postoperative nausea and vomiting (PONV). The latter is highly relevant if the patient is being treated as a day case as it may delay discharge from the unit or even require overnight admission if protracted. Recent work has demonstrated no deleterious effects of nitrous oxide on bowel distension during laparoscopic cholecystectomy (Taylor *et al.* 1992) and the effects on PONV have been vigorously disputed in the anaesthetic literature (Watcha & White 1992, Hartung 1993).

Fluid replacement

Hypotension is a frequent accompaniment to laparoscopy, especially if performed in the head-up position, and occurs more commonly during laparoscopic than during conventional cholecystectomy (Rose *et al.* 1992). Adequate fluid replacement reduces the incidence of hypotension (Fishburne & Keith 1977).

During laparoscopy, blood loss is difficult to assess, as only a small area of the surgical field is visible at any time. Classical signs of occult bleeding such as hypotension, tachycardia and reduction in urine output (if measured) are unreliable during anaesthesia. A high index of suspicion and frequent inspection of the peritoneal cavity by the surgeon are necessary if bleeding is suspected and appropriate volume replacement instituted.

Monitoring

Cardiography

ECG monitoring is mandatory during any procedure under general anaesthesia. Dysrhythmias are particularly common during laparoscopy, primarily because of the effects of hypercarbia and associated catecholamine secretion potentiating the effects of halothane on the heart. The introduction of neuromuscular blocking drugs with little vagolytic action, (e.g. atracurium and vecuronium) together with potent opioids (e.g. fentanyl) increase the likelihood of bradycardia during laparoscopy.

Noninvasive blood pressure (NIBP)

Pneumoperitoneum and head-up tilt (as during laparoscopic cholecystectomy) reduce cardiac performance, so a fall in blood pressure must be anticipated (Rose *et al.* 1992, Noirot *et al.* 1992). Other causes of cardiovascular collapse and hypotension are noted in the section on haemodynamics. Automatic NIBP measurements must be made at frequent intervals (5 minutes or less).

Pulse oximetry

Hypoxaemia is a common accompaniment to laparoscopy due to pre-existing lung pathology, equipment failure and poor anaesthetic technique (e.g. oesophageal or endobronchial intubation), hypoventilation, intrapulmonary shunting and reduced cardiac output (Cunningham & Schlanger 1992). Continuous monitoring of arterial oxygen saturation is mandatory at all times, from induction of anaesthesia until full patient recovery has occurred.

Capnography

End-tidal monitoring of carbon dioxide tension is necessary for determining optimum ventilation rate and depth for the patient who is mechanically ventilated. It is closely related to arterial carbon dioxide tensions during laparoscopy (McKinstry *et al.* 1992). Simple calculation of minute volume from standard charts is inadequate during prolonged insufflation of carbon dioxide, as absorption of gas through the peritoneum adds significantly to carbon dioxide levels in the blood in some patients. In patients who are allowed to breathe spontaneously, a raised end-tidal carbon dioxide tension suggests the need to ventilate.

Temperature

During procedures lasting more than one hour (e.g. lymphadenectomy and nephrectomy), naso-pharyngeal temperature must be monitored. Rectal temperature may not give an accurate representation of core temperature during pneumoperitoneum. Body temperature falls after induction of anaesthesia, as warmer core blood distributes to the cooler periphery. This is due to inhibition of neurones in the preoptic hypothalamic nuclei (POH) which also control the body's response to thermal stress. General anaesthetics such as halothane, together with opioids such as fentanyl, depress the threshold for vasoconstriction under anaesthesia by 2–3°C.

By promoting peripheral vasodilation, inhalational anaesthetics increase heat loss by radiation, conduction and evaporation. The use of neuromuscular blockers inhibits heat production by abolition of shivering (Green 1993). Active measures must be taken to maintain body heat, such as humidification of inspired gases, warming blankets, keeping the operating theatre warm (21–23°C) and warming all fluids given intravenously. Previous anecdotal evidence suggested that the cold insufflating gas also contributed to reducing patient temperature. However, our studies using intra-abdominal thermistors during laparoscopic procedures have shown that the intra-abdominal temperature only fluctuates close to the CO_2 entry port and that over 5 cm away the temperature is maintained within 1°C despite flows of up to 700 l of CO_2 (M.J. Coptcoat & M. Matuszewski, personal communication).

Invasive monitoring of central venous and arterial pressure

Invasive monitoring of central venous and arterial pressure is desirable for those procedures, such as laparoscopic nephrectomy and cystectomy, where blood loss rarely but realistically can be considerable and there is a delay in even immediate open exploration.

Patient position

Great care should be taken to ensure the patient pressure points are well padded during prolonged procedures to prevent skin and nerve ischaemia. In addition, the steep head-down tilt sometimes necessary for bowel displacement during lymphadenectomy requires that a non-slip mattress be used on the operating table.

Insufflating gases

The insufflating gas must be:
nonirritant
nonflammable (as diathermy is frequently used)
soluble in blood (to minimize the effects of inadvertent intravascular injection)
cost-effective.

Although air was used initially, it is 20 times less soluble than carbon dioxide, so the results of inadvertent intravascular injection would be catastrophic. It also supports combustion.

Nitrous oxide has been advocated by some as it is nearly as soluble as carbon dioxide, it does not impose a CO_2 load (Corrall *et al.* 1974) and causes less peritoneal irritation (Uhlich 1982). However, it can form explosive mixtures in combination with methane gas escaping through the bowel wall, so its use has been abandoned in those cases where a diathermy must be used. Nevertheless, it remains popular for diagnostic procedures carried out under local anaesthetic (Uhlich 1982).

Carbon dioxide has been found, overall, to be the most satisfactory gas for insufflation. Doubts have been expressed concerning the extent of CO_2 absorption from the peritoneal cavity. Seed *et al.* (1970) did not find it a problem in patients who were mechanically ventilated and considered the amount absorbed to be small. Nevertheless, Hodgson *et al.* (1970) found it sufficiently large to recommend mechanical ventilation in patients undergoing laparoscopy. By measurement of both oxygen uptake and carbon dioxide production using a metabolic computer, Blobner *et al.* (1992) have confirmed an increase in carbon dioxide uptake during laparoscopic cholecystectomy. In one case, the accidental production of subcutaneous CO_2 emphysema resulted in a marked increase in $V\text{CO}_2$ and a raised $Pa\text{CO}_2$ despite an increase in minute ventilation to $200\,\text{ml}\,\text{kg}^{-1}\,\text{min}^{-1}$. Blobner *et al.* also confirmed that higher intra-abdominal pressures protect against further absorption of gas by compressing the venous capillaries of the peritoneum.

The reason for these different results is due to the fact that carbon dioxide absorption from the peritoneum is a complex interaction between:

volume and tension of gas insufflated
solubility of the gas in blood
escape into the tissue (causing emphysema)
perfusion of the cavity walls (and the consequent ability of the venous drainage to transport the gas into the portal or systemic circulation).

Given the variation in amount of gas insufflated, intracavity pressure and venous drainage, it is not surprising that differences have been found in CO_2 uptake. As far as inadvertent CO_2 embolism is concerned, it is reassuring to note that radiologists have rapidly injected 50–100 ml of carbon dioxide for cardiac contrast studies with no ill effects (Lewis *et al.* 1972). Up to 7.5 ml kg^{-1} of CO_2 has been tolerated intravenously whereas only 0.25 ml kg^{-1} has proven lethal in cats (Yacoub *et al.* 1982). The rapidity with which CO_2 is excreted by the lungs and absorbed into the body stores makes it the safest gas at present in use.

Pathophysiological effects of laparoscopy

Haemodynamic

The haemodynamic effects of laparoscopy extend from minor hypotensive episodes requiring no specific treatment to cardiac arrest. They are the result of a complex interaction between the following:

- Patient position can cause a decrease in venous return, being particularly noted where a pronounced head-up tilt is used. In addition to general anaesthesia and mechanical ventilation, this can result in a marked reduction in cardiac output, although blood pressure is usually maintained by an increase in systemic vascular resistance (Noirot *et al.* 1992).
- Hypoventilation because of a head-down position or absorption of carbon dioxide leads to hypercarbia which can induce dysrhythmias and a fall in cardiac output (Fishburne & Keith 1977).
- Blood loss, as in any surgical procedure, causes reduced venous return and reduced cardiac output.
- Perforation of a major vessel or viscus by a trocar can occur prior to insertion of the laparoscope and may go unnoticed initially.
- Traction or stimulation of visceral peritoneum may induce a vasovagal response, resulting in bradycardia and even cardiac arrest (Fishburne & Keith 1977). This can be prevented by the use of vagolytic drugs, such as atropine.

Gas embolus is one of the most feared complications of laparoscopy but it is fortunately an extremely rare complication (Phillips *et al.* 1976). Signs of gas embolus include hypotension, cardiac dysrhythmias, a fall in oxygen saturation and cardiac arrest. The presence of a 'mill wheel' murmur over the precordium is suggestive, but the only absolute criterion is the presence of gas in the circulation. Differential diagnosis of cardiac collapse includes any of the above causes, but if gas embolus is suspected urgent measures must be taken.

Since cardiac output is impeded by the compressible pocket of gas which usually ends up in the right ventricular outflow tract, these measures include immediate cessation of insufflation, turning the patient on the left side in a slight head-down position and aspiration of air from the right ventricle following insertion of a central venous catheter (Yacoub *et al.* 1982). The latter should not be necessary with carbon dioxide as the insufflating gas as it is rapidly absorbed into the blood stream.

It is sensible to administer 100% oxygen during this time as hypoxaemia is certain to be an accompaniment. If the gas enters visceral veins then air may be trapped in the portal circulation and this can result in delayed death from gas embolism.

Is laparoscopy safer for the cardiac or haemodynamically compromised patient than an equivalent open procedure? Few studies have directly addressed this aspect although a recent examination of the cardiovascular changes associated with a raised intra-abdominal pressure (due to insufflation) concluded that the 'haemodynamic changes produced could be deleterious in patients with compromised cardiac function' (Noirot *et al.*1992).

Hypotension was found to be a 'common problem' during laparoscopic cholecystectomy versus open in a retrospective case note study (Rose *et al.* 1992).

Respiratory

Hypercapnoea

Many early studies concentrated on the adverse effects of patient position (head-down) and raised IAP causing a reduction in minute volume. This led to recommendations to ventilate the patient (Seed *et al.*, Hodgson *et al.* 1970). During shorter procedures in slim patients, spontaneous ventilation using a face mask is acceptable and does not lead to significant hypercarbia, acidosis or cardiac arrhythmias (Kenefick *et al.* 1987).

Diaphragmatic function is compromised both by raised IAP and the full weight of the viscera being borne by the diaphragm in the head-down position. In addition, the fall in functional residual capacity causes an increased shunt and subsequent hypoxaemia (Fishburne & Keith 1977).

Absorption of gases, particularly carbon dioxide, may lead to hypoxaemia and hypercapnoea as stated earlier, continuing after cessation of insufflation and even into the early postoperative period (Lewis *et al.* 1972).

Hypoxaemia

The differential diagnosis of hypoxaemia during laparoscopy includes pre-existing conditions such as respiratory disease, hypoventilation, increased shunting due to such conditions as endobronchial intubation, pneumothorax, subcutaneous emphysema and aspiration of gastric contents, and reduced cardiac output. During laparoscopy, some or all of these factors may be sufficiently severe to preclude adequate oxygenation (i.e. maintenance of oxygen saturation above 90%) and to force abandonment in favour of an open procedure when oxygenation is immediately restored to normal (Cunningham & Schlanger 1992).

Pneumothorax

Pneumothorax may occur during any surgical procedure; that specifically due to laparoscopy may occur as a result of defects in the embryological development of the diaphragm.

The posterior, lateral and central portions are formed by the fusion of the dorsal mesentery and mesoderm with the pleuroperitoneal membrane. This membrane is derived from the pulmonary ridge, so if the mesoderm is not properly deposited at any of these adjacent points of union, a failure of proper fusion may result in congenital diaphragmatic defects.

Increased IAP from insufflation could force gas from the peritoneal to the pleural space. The higher IAP needs to be, in order to produce an adequate pneumoperitoneum, the greater the likelihood of significant pneumothorax in susceptible patients. Reduction of IAP is best achieved by full relaxation of the abdominal wall with specific neuromuscular blocking drugs. In addition, using carbon dioxide as the insufflating gas ensures rapid removal of the gas from the pleural cavity (Doctor & Hussain 1973).

Gastrointestinal

It is commonly supposed that laparoscopy increases the likelihood of regurgitation of gastric contents due to a combination of head-down tilt and raised IAP. In fact, the risk may be much smaller than previously thought, as raised IAP may actually *increase* the pressure of the lower oesophageal sphincter and thus limit regurgitation (Jones *et al.* 1989).

A prospective series of 50,048 laparoscopies studied by a working party indicated only one case of aspiration and this occurred at induction of anaesthesia, an incidence of 0.002% (Chamberlain & Carron Brown 1978). This is much less than the 2% incidence reported by Duffy (1979). Roberts & Goodman (1990) used a pH electrode positioned just above the gastro-oesophageal junction and were unable to demonstrate acid reflux in any of the patients studied. (Note that reflux of acid into the lower oesophagus is not synonymous with acid regurgitation into the lungs.) They concluded that endotracheal intubation is not justified on the grounds of airway protection alone but may be required for the other reasons stated above.

Postoperative effects and complications

Pain

Reduction in surgical trauma in laparoscopic versus open procedures should result in a reduction of postoperative pain, lessened requirement for opioids and earlier return to normal activity.

In a retrospective study of 189 major laparoscopic procedures (101 laparoscopic versus 88 conventional cholecystectomies) there was a statistically significant reduction in excessive pain (4% vs. 12%, $P<0.05$) and narcotic requirement (67% vs 94%, $P<0.01$) in the laparoscopic group (Rose *et al.* 1992).

In an effort to reduce the opioid requirement still further, non-steroidal anti-inflammatory drugs (NSAIDs) have been administered along with conventional opioids on demand. Ketorolac is a popular NSAID in this regard, which can be given intravenously at induction of anaesthesia. When used in this way opioid requirements are reduced in the postoperative period (Liu *et al.* 1992). We have found that the routine use of local anaesthesia (bupivicaine 0.5%) in the port wounds almost abolishes any memory of a laparoscopic procedure in our day-case unit.

Myalgias

Vague shoulder-tip pain, neck stiffness and muscle pains, nausea and headache are common accompaniments to laparoscopy (Kenefick *et al.* 1987). Escape of gas from the peritoneal cavity into the pleural cavity with irritation of the visceral pleura is the presumed cause. Although the exact mechanism is unknown, neck pain and stiffness can be reduced by avoiding suxamethonium as the relaxant (Smith *et al.* 1992).

Nausea and vomiting

Nausea and vomiting are common accompaniments to laparoscopy, especially gynaecological. However, it is doubtful whether it is more common following a procedure carried out laparoscopically versus the equivalent open operation. Rose *et al.* (1992) found a similar incidence of nausea and vomiting in patients receiving open versus laparoscopic cholecystectomy. Unfortunately, increased use of NSAIDs in place of opioids has not resulted in a reduction in this unpleasant side-effect (Liu *et al.* 1992).

Respiratory function

Major reductions in peak expiratory flow rate (PEFR), forced expiratory volume in 1 second (FEV_1) and forced vital capacity (FVC) are seen after upper abdominal surgery. It is presumed that replacement of a major (painful) abdominal incision by multiple small ones would produce an improvement in lung function.

This would be particularly appropriate for patients with pre-existing lung pathology who are at high risk of developing upper respiratory tract infection. In a study of 20 patients randomly assigned to laparoscopic or open cholecystectomy, Putensen-Himmer *et al.* (1992) showed that respiratory function is less impaired and recovery improved. For instance, at 24 hours post-surgery FEV_1 in the laparoscopic group was 85% of control versus 54% in the open group.

Minimizing deterioration in postoperative lung function by using laparoscopic versus open cholecystectomy (or nephrectomy) has obvious advantages for patients with pre-existing respiratory dysfunction or those in whom oxygen desaturation *must* be avoided in the post-operative period; for example, patients with sickle cell disease (Davenport *et al.* 1991). However, less convincing differences were seen by Gögler *et al.* (1992) who found a high degree of pulmonary dysfunction in both groups.

Discharge from hospital versus open procedures

No studies have prospectively documented the difference in length of hospital study in laparoscopic versus open procedures, e.g. nephrectomy. Rose *et al.* (1992) looked at hospital outcome in a retrospective comparison and found a significant reduction in hospital stay for laparoscopic (2.5 days) versus open cholecystectomy (6.6. days, $P<0.001$). It would appear that the increased cost of surgical time can be offset by reduced length of hospital stay.

References

Blobner M., Felber A.R., Gögler S., Weigl E.M., Jelen-Esselhorn S. (1992) Carbon dioxide uptake from pneumoperitoneum during laparoscopic cholecystectomy. *Anesthesiology*, **77**, A37.

Chamberlain G.V.P., Carron Brown J.A. eds (1978) Gynaecological laparoscopy: The report of the working party of the confidential enquiry into gynaecological laparoscopy. The Royal College of Obstetricians and Gynaecologists, London.

Corrall I.M., Knights K., Potter D.R., Strunin L. (1974) Arterial oxygen tension during laparoscopy with nitrous oxide in the spontaneously breathing patient. *British Journal of Anaesthesia*, **46**, 925–8.

Cunningham A.J., Schlanger M. (1992) Intraoperative hypoxemia complicating laparoscopic cholecystectomy in a patient with sickle hemoglobinopathy. *Anesthesia Annals*, **75**, 838–43.

Davenport M., Howard E.R., Green D.W. (1991) Minimally invasive surgery in sickle cell disease. *British Medical Journal*, **303**, 249.

Doctor N.H. & Hussain Z. (1973) Bilateral pneumothorax associated with laparoscopy. *Anaesthesia*, **28**, 75–81.

Duffy B.L. (1979) Regurgitation during pelvic laparoscopy. *British Journal of Anaesthesia*, **51**, 1089–90.

Eger E.I. II, Saidman L.J. (1965) Hazards of nitrous oxide anesthesia in bowel obstruction and pneumothorax. *Anesthesiology*, **26**, 61–6.

Fishburne J.I., Keith L. (1977) Anesthesia. In *Laparoscopy* (ed. J.M. Phillips), pp.69–85. Williams and Wilkins, Baltimore.

Gögler S., Felber A.R., Blobner M., Laubrock I., Jelen-Esselhorn S. (1992) Pulmonary function following laparoscopic cholecystectomy versus laparotomic cholecystectomy. *Anesthesiology*, **77**, A10.

Green D.W. (1993) Anaesthesia for microvascular surgery. In *Anaesthesia for Burns, Maxillofacial and Plastic Surgery* (ed. H. Patel), pp.101–2. Edward Arnold, London.

Hartung J. (1993) Nitrous oxide—It's enough to make you vomit. *Anesthesiology*, **78**, 403–5.

Hodgson C., McClelland R.M.A., Newton J.R. (1970) Some effects of the peritoneal insufflation of carbon dioxide at laparoscopy. *Anaesthesia*, **25**, 382–90.

Jones M.J., Mitchell R.W., Hindocha N. (1989) Effect of increased intra-abdominal pressure during laparoscopy on the lower oesophageal sphincter. *Anesthesia Annals*, **68**, 63–5.

Kenefick J.P., Leader A., Maltby J.R., Taylor P.J. (1987) Laparoscopy: blood gas values and minor sequelae associated with three techniques based on isoflurane. *British Journal of Anaesthesia*, **59**, 189–94.

Lewis D.G., Ryder W., Burn N., Wheldon J.T., Tacchi D. (1972) Laparoscopy—an investigation during spontaneous ventilation with halothane. *British Journal of Anaesthesia*, **44**, 685–90.

Liu J., Ding Y., White P.F., Feinstein R., Shear J. (1992) Laparoscopic cholecystectomy: effect of ketorolac on postoperative pain and ventilatory function. *Anesthesiology*, **77**, A1255.

Marco A.P., Yeo C.J., Rock P. (1990) Anesthesia for patients undergoing laparoscopic cholecystectomy. *Anesthesiology*, **73**, 168–170.

McKinstry L.J., Perverseff R.A., Yip R.W. (1992) Arterial and end-tidal carbon dioxide in patients undergoing laparoscopic cholecystectomy. *Anesthesiology*, **77**, A108.

Noirot D., Joris J., Legrand M., Lamy M. (1992) Hemodynamic changes during pneumoperitoneum for laparoscopic cholecystectomy. *Anesthesiology*, **77**, A69.

Phillips J.M., Keith D., Hulka J., Hulka B., Keith L. (1976) Gynecologic laparoscopy in 1975. *Journal of Reproductive Medicine*, **16**, 105-17.

Putensen-Himmer G., Putensen C., Lammer H., Lingnau W., Aigner F., Benzer H. (1992) Comparison of postoperative respiratory function after laparoscopy or open laparotomy for cholecystectomy. *Anesthesiology*, **77**: 4, 675-80.

Roberts C.J., Goodman N.W. (1990) Gastro-oesophageal reflux during elective laparoscopy. *Anaesthesia*, **45**, 1009–11.

Rose D.K.R., Cohen M.M., Soutter D.I. (1992) Laparoscopic cholecystectomy: the anaesthetist's point of view. *Canadian Journal of Anaesthesia*, **39**, 809–15.

Seed R.F., Shakespeare T.F., Muldoon M.J. (1970) Carbon dioxide homeostasis during anaesthesia for laparoscopy. *Anaesthesia*, **25**, 223–31.

Smith I., Ding Y., White P.F. (1992) Post-laparoscopic myalgias: effect of propofol, succinycholine and atracurium. *Anesthesiology*, **77**, A951.

Taylor E., Feinstein R., White P.F., Soper N. (1992) Anaesthesia for laparoscopic cholecystectomy. Is nitrous oxide contraindicated? *Anesthesiology*, **76**, 541–3.

Uhlich G.A. (1982) Laparoscopy: the question of the proper gas. *Gastrointestinal Endoscopy*, **28**, 212–13.

Watcha M.F., White P.F. (1992) Post-operative nausea and vomiting. *Anesthesiology*, **77**, 162–84.

Yacoub O.F., Cardona I., Coveler L.A., Dodson M.G. (1982) Carbon dioxide embolism during laparoscopy. *Anesthesiology*, **57**, 533-535.

6: Complications of Laparoscopy

M.J. COPTCOAT AND A.D. JOYCE

Introduction

Operative laparoscopy is minimally invasive and is associated with a low morbidity and rapid return to normal activities. But complications, although infrequent, can occur at any point of a laparoscopic procedure. The majority are minor and do not drastically alter the outcome, but on some rare occasions a minimally invasive concept is transformed into a maximally invasive emergency salvage procedure. Prevention is better than cure, and fortunately most complications can be nipped in the bud by the alert laparoscopist.

The complications of a laparoscopic cholecystectomy have been much discussed recently, and the stark fact is that common bile duct injury (and, in particular, stricture formation) during a laparoscopic cholecystectomy is many times more common than was seen following an open cholecystectomy. The conclusion is not that the procedure is inherently dangerous but that surgeons have not been adequately trained (Peters *et al.* 1991).

Before a resumé of possible laparoscopic complications and their management, let us focus on prevention, which in retrospect comes from adequate training. Operative laparoscopy is a quantum leap from even modern endourology, and experience needs to be gained with simulators and, ideally, *in vivo* rehearsal before patients are treated. Many laparoscopic procedures in urology follow the same basic protocol, especially techniques in the pelvis. There is, then, an overlap and consolidation of experience. But more advanced procedures such as a laparoscopic nephrectomy or pyeloplasty need specific training, and some form of preceptorship is preferred if early complications are to be kept to a minimum.

Two characteristics of laparoscopy in urology stand out at the present time. The first is that the surgeon's age is often inversely proportional to the surgeon's laparoscopic acumen and, second, our trainees have to learn from relatively inexperienced senior staff. Our gynaecological colleagues who have been immersed in laparoscopy, albeit mainly of the simple variety, do not have the same problems. Their advice to us is to overtrain through this chronological problem and we will witness future urologists just as adept at laparoscopy as at transurethral resection or open bladder reconstruction. Until this time, centres that specialize in laparoscopic work will continue to be the focus of work and training. But in one generation, the full breadth of laparoscopy in urology will be seen in every urology department.

It is too early in the development and learning of these new operative laparoscopic procedures to know the true incidence of complications. At the present time we can only look at a comparison with previous laparoscopic work in gynaecology (Table 6.1), with the cautionary note that most complications occur when the laparoscopic surgeon has performed fewer than 250 procedures. We are optimistic that this is not a figure to be highlighted in urology, because the instrumentation is safer, and we know from video TURP studies that the learning curve of an operator when he is constantly viewed is much more rapid.

The incidence of gynaecological laparoscopic-related morbidity is estimated to be less than 4% (Mintz 1977, Kane & Kreijs 1984). A summary of the morbidity in our first 150 cases at King's College Hospital appears in Table 6.2. Its urological total of 10% sits uncomfortably beside the previous gynaecological total of under 4%, but it includes a series of 43 laparoscopic nephrectomy cases. If this special group is excluded, the incidence of complications falls to 5.8%. Of our total complications for all laparoscopic procedures, only three cases were abandoned peroperatively. Two were for nonprogression of laparoscopic nephrectomies due to dense inflammatory adhesions associated with stone disease, and a third was a laparoscopic node dissection that had to be opened to control a bleeding point. Four cases of postoperative haemorrhage occurred after laparoscopic nephrectomies. These patients were explored with a laparotomy 4–12 hours postoperatively because of a fall in haemoglobin and a persistent tachycardia. Blood loss from a wound drain was not a reliable sign and it was disappointing to note that after completion of each of these laparoscopic nephrectomies, good haemostasis had been observed. Our feeling is that occult haemorrhage can occur below a thin puddle of clotted blood, and so meticulous irrigation, aspiration and, if necessary, swabbing of the renal bed are required before removing the ports.

Further specific complications will be covered in each procedure later in this book. General complications and their management will now be discussed.

Table 6.1 Incidence of complications of gynaecological laparoscopy (Phillips 1977)

Complication	Incidence %
Pneumoperitoneum-related	0.7
Haemorrhage	0.6
Perforating injuries	0.3
Infection	0.1
Intestinal burns	0.05
Cardiac arrest	0.03
Total	1.78

Table 6.2 Complications of laparoscopic urological surgery in 150 cases at King's College Hospital, London

Complication	Incidence	
Access		
Pneumoperitoneum		7
Perforating injuries	(4.6%)	
		0
Operative		
Haemorrhage		
Cardiac dysrhythmia		1
	(0.6%)	
Postoperative		1
Local infections	(0.6%)	
Chest infections		
Urinary retention		
Haemorrhage		0
		2
Total	(1.2%)	

Problems with access

Pneumoperitoneum

The choice of gases for establishing a pneumoperitoneum and the complications of carbon dioxide insufflation have been mentioned in Chapter 5.

The complications of Veress needle and trocar insertion have been greatly reduced by the use of disposable ports and needles with safety shields. An unusual complication of insufflation needle placement is massive distention of the preperitoneal space when the tip of the needle has not gone through into the peritoneum. This should be suspected if the injection of 5 ml of saline meets with resistance and initial insufflation pressures stay at the upper predetermined limit of 12 mmHg. Recognition of this problem sometimes only occurs with the introduction of the laparoscope. In these cases, the Veress needle should be inserted lateral to the rectus sheath, and similarly the first port should be placed well away from the now artificially thickened central abdominal wall. Initial intraperitoneal views will still seem cramped but this will disappear as the carbon dioxide is absorbed.

Abdomens that have undergone previous surgery or where one suspects intraperitoneal adhesions must be respected, and if there is any doubt that a free intra-abdominal space cannot be entered then an open minilaparotomy incision should be made and the first cannula with blunt trocar inserted as described by Hasson (1971). Subsequent port sitings can then be made under direct vision after preliminary adhesions have been divided. Routine placement of the first port in this way is recommended for those inexperienced in using a Veress needle, and it would certainly avoid the rare but catastrophic aortic perforation incident (Peterson *et al.* 1982).

Insufflation of carbon dioxide into the peritoneal cavity is sometimes associated with postoperative shoulder pain. This referred pain is believed to be the result of direct irritation of the diaphragm by carbon dioxide forming carbonic acid. It may occur in as many as one-third of patients, but is usually severe in fewer than 5%. Slow initial insufflation helps to reduce the complication but, if present, generally it will resolve spontaneously within 24 hours. Prolonged operative laparoscopic procedures are also associated with widespread surgical emphysema if the seals around the ports are not secure. Although dramatic, this is usually completely asymptomatic, but nurses and junior medical staff should be aware of its unimportant presence. It is exaggerated during and after laparoscopic pelvic lymphadenectomy with the formation of a pneumocele of the scrotum.

Trocar placement

A potential complication of trocar placement is a vascular injury within the abdominal wall. This may result in bleeding around the cannula and into the peritoneal cavity or the formation of an abdominal wall haematoma. The abdominal wall should be transilluminated with the laparoscope before incising the skin and inserting the trocar. If an arterial or venous injury does occur then the cannula should be left in place to tamponade the vessel and allow it to seal. All trocar insertion sites should be carefully examined prior to and after removal of the cannula.

If active bleeding is identified (this is usually from the superficial epigastric artery), a haemostatic suture can be placed with a hand needle through the abdominal wall or by passage of a Stamey needle under laparoscopic vision (Green *et al.* 1992).

The risk of a trocar injury to the gastrointestinal tract is very small in the absence of dense adhesions. However, bowel preparations are recommended during difficult cases when the bowel must be retracted in order for the surgeon to operate accurately. Gastrointestinal (Soderstrom & Levy 1986), vascular (Lynn *et al.* 1982) or urinary tract injuries (Deshmukh 1982) resulting from laparoscopic trocar insertion are rare (0.3%) and should be managed in the same way as any other penetrating injury to the abdomen.

Injury from an insufflation needle to a major blood vessel is unlikely to require an immediate laparotomy, providing that pressure can be applied from an associate blunt instrument. However, unlike insufflation-needle injuries, perforation of a major blood vessel with a trocar should be managed by immediate laparotomy and repair.

If the abdomen does need to be opened in an emergency, a safe but rapid technique is to pull the laparoscope up against the abdominal wall and cut down into it with a skin knife.

Endocoordination

Endocoordination is an important aspect of the laparoscopic surgical learning curve. The two-dimensional image produced by current laparoscopic video systems results in a loss of depth perception. This handicap can be partially overcome by adapting specific visual clues to assist in the proper placement and orientation of laparoscopic instruments. It is important to maintain continual visualization of the operating instruments on the video monitor. When the telescope is removed, all instruments should be kept stationary. It is this relative lack of depth perception that requires a long learning curve.

For the assistant, whose orientation is at 180° to the telescope and camera, the visual problem may be compounded by a monitor with a seemingly inverted image. The critical angle of a manipulation instrument to the field of vision is 90°. Anything less than 90°, and especially close to being parallel, proves to be easy, but an angle over 90° is a very difficult hand–brain challenge. If the problem is not artificially corrected on the monitor, assistants must consciously think about what they are doing rather than what it appears they may have to do with their instruments. Some find it easier to view the surgeon's monitor regardless of the position difficulties.

The bowel may be injured by diathermy, either directly or, very rarely, as a complication of capacitance discharge via a metal cannula that is insulated from the abdominal wall by a nonconductive grip. It is sometimes difficult to locate the exact point, and if injury is suspected, careful and gradual inspection from a standard reference point such as the caecum should be carried out, and any bowel injury should be oversewn. This can easily be accomplished with modern needle-holders and sutures.

Haemorrhage

The greatest problem facing laparoscopic surgeons is haemorrhage. It is rarely so severe as to require an emergency laparotomy, but on many occasions what might have been a trivial leak corrected by tamponade can produce an inoperative field. First, the bleeding tends to obscure the line of dissection. Second, blood absorbs light intensity with consequent reduction in vision. Attempted aspiration of blood can inadvertently remove the carbon dioxide from the operative space, and so it collapses. This in turn allows more blood to ooze, and what should have been a minor complication can lead to an unnecessary open laparotomy. Prevention is by anticipating any bleeding with the use of grasping forceps close to the site of dissection.

Any potential haemorrhage can be grasped by either the operator or the assistant. Then there is plenty of time to exchange instruments for either a clip applier or diathermy. The important practical point about applying clips is that one should always be able to see the ends approximate on the other side of the vessel. If a position cannot be identified then one must suspect that haemostasis will not be intact. Siting of the clip ends is also important to determine that they have not crept onto another associated structure. Many of the common bile duct injuries during a laparoscopic cholecystectomy have been due to misplacement of haemostatic clips.

References

Deshmukh A.S. (1982) Laparoscopic bladder injury. *Urology*, **19**, 306–7.

Green L.S., Loughlin K.R., Kavoussi L.R. (1992) Management of epigastric vessel injury during laparoscopy. *Journal of Endourology*, **6**: 2, 99-101.

Hasson H.M. (1971) A modified instrument and method for laparoscopy. *American Journal of Obstetrics and Gynaecolgy*, **110**: 6, 886–7.

Kane M.G., Kreijs G.J. (1984) Complications of diagnostic laparoscopy in Dallas: A seven-year prospective study. *Gastrointestinal Endoscopy*, **30**, 237–40.

Lynn S.C., Katz A.R., Ross P.J. (1982) Aortic perforation sustained at laparoscopy. *Journal of Reproductive Medicine*, **27**, 217–19.

Mintz M. (1977) Risks and prophylaxis in laparoscopy: A survey of 100,000 cases. *Journal of Reproductive Medicine*, **18**, 269–72.

Peters J.H., Ellison E.C., Innes J.T. *et al.* (1991) Safety and efficacy of laparoscopic cholecystectomy. *Annals of Surgery*, **213**, 3-12.

Peterson H.B., Greenspan J.R., Ory H.W. (1982) Death following puncture of the aorta during laparoscopic sterilization. *Obstetrics and Gynaecology*, **59**, 133–4.

Phillips J.M. (1977) Complications in laparoscopy. *International Journal of Gynaecology and Obstetrics*, **15**, 157–62.

Soderstrom R.M., Levy B.S. (1986) Bowel injuries during laparoscopy: Causes and medicolegal questions. *Continuing Obstetrics and Gynaecology*, **27**, 41-45.

7: The Metabolic Response to Operative Laparoscopy

C. G. EDEN AND M. J. COPTCOAT

Introduction

The explosion of interest in operative laparoscopy by surgeons and the public alike has resulted in an almost unique event in surgical history. With the notable exception of extracorporeal shockwave lithotripsy, no other treatment modality has been so widely and rapidly embraced without having first proven its safety and superiority in comparative clinical trials. There seems to be an intuitive feeling amongst the surgical fraternity, hitherto based largely on anecdotal evidence, that an operation performed through a small hole must somehow be better for the patient.

Balanced against the potential benefit of this minimal-access approach is the longer anaesthetic time for many laparoscopic operations, especially for complex procedures such as nephrectomy and ureterolysis. This is of concern, because we already know from sham operations on animals that a general anaesthetic alone elicits a stress response and from human studies that anaesthesia causes immune compromise (Platt *et al.* 1989).

The economic benefits of a laparoscopic approach in the context of gallbladder surgery are well established (Cuschieri *et al.* 1990): it allows an earlier discharge from hospital and return to work, in addition to a smaller postoperative analgesic requirement. However, little attention has been paid to determining how operative laparoscopy compares with open surgery at the biological level.

The metabolic response to trauma

Evolutionary selection pressures undoubtedly conferred some advantage on those seriously injured ancestors of ours whose metabolism could mobilize energy stores and retain water to aid healing whilst they were unable to forage.

An identical metabolic response is seen after modern surgery, but we now recognize that the hyperglycaemia, negative nitrogen balance, fluid retention and muscle weakness that result can be harmful, particularly in patients with little cardiorespiratory or nutritional reserve. The accompanying relative immunosupression leads to an increased susceptibility to exogenous and nosocomial infection (Chandra 1983), impaired wound-healing and tissue repair (Windsor *et al.* 1988) and, more worryingly, may adversely affect the results of surgery for malignancy.

Table 7.1 Mediators of the stress response (Wilmore 1991)

Hormone	Cytokine	Lipid
Glucagon	Tumour necrosis factor	Platelet-activating factor
Glucocorticoids	Interleukin-1 Interleukin-2 Thromboxane A2 Interleukin-6	
Catecholamines	Interferon gamma	Leucotriene B4
Arginine vasopressin	Prostaglandin E2	
Aldosterone		

Mediators of the stress response

The mediators of the stress response can be divided into three groups: hormones, cytokines and lipid mediators (Table 7.1). The pattern of mediator release depends on the stressful stimulus applied, and it appears that the three response systems are interconnected by amplification loops and negative-feedback systems (Wilmore 1991).

The role of carbon dioxide

The ready availability, low cost and inertness of carbon dioxide (CO_2) has made it the gas of choice for the creation and maintenance of a pneumoperitoneum. Its disadvantage lies in its great solubility in peritoneal fluid, forming carbonic acid. Intraoperative and early postoperative pooling of carbonic acid under the diaphragm and consequent diaphragmatic irritation is thought to be responsible for the postlaparoscopy pain syndrome, which is characterized by shoulder-tip pain.

The pain is more commonly felt on the right, probably due to trapping of fluid between the liver and the right hemidiaphragm. The chief practical problem caused by the great solubility of CO_2, however, is the generation of a metabolic acidosis caused by absorption of carbonic acid, even when the intraperitoneal pressure is continuously maintained below 12mmHg.

This can lead to cardiac dysrhythmias and depression of cardiac output, and occasionally it necessitates conversion to an open procedure. Continuous monitoring of end-tidal CO_2 ($EtCO_2$) is therefore essential as it may be necessary to increase the minute-volume ventilation to maintain the $EtCO_2$ in the ideal range of 4.5–5.5%. This is particularly so during relatively long laparoscopic procedures such as nephrectomy.

The evidence presented by clinical studies

The hypothesis that it is less metabolically stressful to perform an operation with minimal trauma of access is an attractive one and is the basis for three recent studies which have sought to compare the metabolic responses to a laparoscopic operation with its open counterpart. Two of the studies have compared laparoscopic with open cholecystectomy and the third (Eden & Coptcoat, submitted for publication) has investigated nephrectomy. In addition, a fourth study (Frazee *et al.* 1991) has compared postoperative lung function in patients undergoing laparoscopic and open cholecystectomy.

Laparoscopic cholecystectomy

McMahon *et al.* (1993) compared laparoscopic cholecystectomy with open cholecystectomy performed through a conventional upper midline incision, whilst Mealy *et al.* (1992) used a 5–7 cm minilaparotomy incision. All patients underwent elective surgery. McMahon's group analysed venous blood taken at regular intervals during the first postoperative week for C-reactive protein, interleukin-6, cortisol, albumin, transferrin, iron, fibrinogen, fibrin degradation products, polymorphonuclear elastase, white cell, neutrophil and lymphocyte count. Twenty-four-hour urine collections were analysed for urea, creatinine, 3-methylhistidine and catecholamines. They found that although there was a wide interpersonal variation in the magnitude of the stress response there was no statistically significant difference between the two groups of 10 patients in any of the parameters measured. Mealy investigated the metabolic response to surgery in 21 patients (10 undergoing laparoscopic and 11 open surgery), in addition to assessing postoperative lung function and pain perception using a linear analogue scale. The metabolic parameters measured were urinary cortisol, vanillylmandelic acid (VMA), metanephrines and nitrogen loss, serum complement component C_3 and C-reactive protein (CRP), full blood count and erythrocyte sedimentation rate (ESR). Lung function was assessed by spirometry, peak-flowmetry and arterial blood gas sampling. Statistically significant differences were seen between the two groups in respect of urinary VMA excretion (higher in the laparoscopic group), ESR and CRP values (higher in the open group). Postoperative lung function tests demonstrated a significantly lower pH and higher $P\text{CO}_2$ in the open group, indicating poorer respiratory performance. The postoperative analgesic requirement was also significantly greater in the open group. In a study of 36 consecutive patients undergoing elective cholecystectomy using either a right subcostal incision (16 patients) or a four-port technique (20 patients), Frazee *et al.* (1991) measured lung function using body plethysmography and a flow-volume loop. The distribution of smokers was roughly equal between the two groups. Lung function tests performed both prior to and 24 hours after surgery showed that all three parameters measured—forced vital capacity (FVC), forced expiratory volume at 1 second (FEV_1) and forced expiratory flow 25–75%)—were significantly higher following surgery in the laparoscopic group.

Laparoscopic nephrectomy

In the authors' still unpublished study, 14 consecutive patients undergoing nephrectomy were studied: seven patients in the open group and seven in the laparoscopic group. Patients in the open group underwent nephrectomy via a loin (six patients) or a subcostal approach (one patient): three patients for benign disease and four for malignancy. In the laparoscopic group a five-port transperitoneal ureter-first technique was used for nephrectomy in all seven patients. This involved a preliminary full-length ipsilateral colonic mobilization. Five patients had benign disease and two had a renal malignancy. Arterial blood was regularly sampled in the first 48 hours following surgery for estimation of white count, glucose and blood gases. Twenty-four-hour urine collections were used to measure urea, cortisol and catecholamine excretion at 0, 24, 48 and 168 hours following surgery. Lung function was assessed by spirometry and peakflowmetry prior to surgery and at 24 and 48 hours following surgery.

As in the patients undergoing cholecystectomy, there was no statistical difference in serum glucose, white cell count or urinary urea excretion between the laparoscopic and open groups. However, in contrast to the cholecystectomy patients, there was a significantly higher and more prolonged cortisol rise in the open cases (Fig. 7.1) and although the urinary adrenalin excretion (Fig. 7.2) was higher in the laparoscopic group at 24 hours, it fell more rapidly and was lower

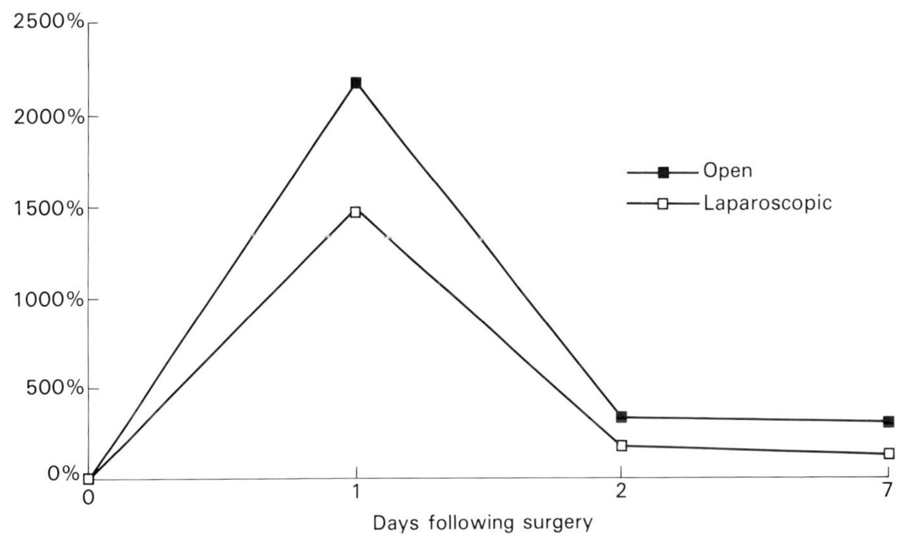

Fig. 7.1 Percentage change in 24-hour urinary cortisol excretion following nephrectomy. There was a significantly higher and more prolonged cortisol rise during an open nephrectomy than a laparoscopic nephrectomy.

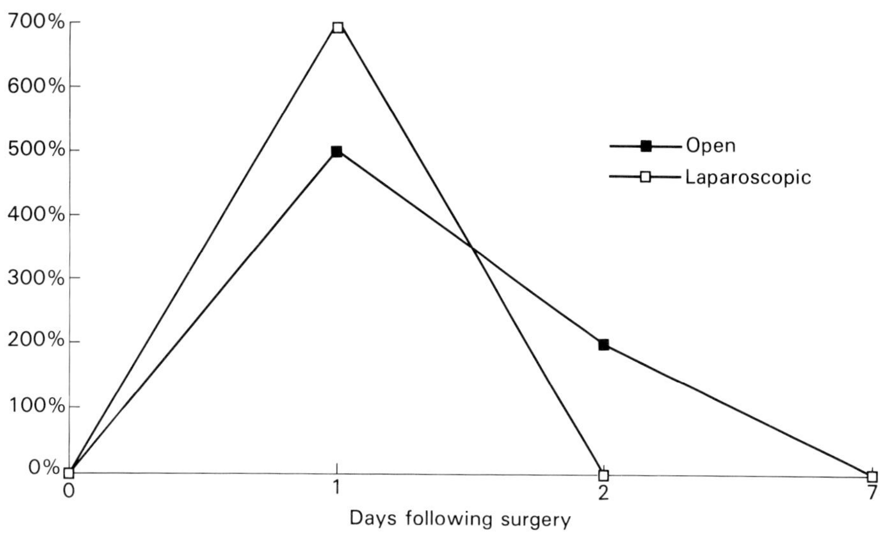

Fig. 7.2 Percentage change in 24-hour urinary adrenalin excretion. The excretion was higher after a laparoscopic nephrectomy until 24 hours postoperatively. Then it fell more rapidly and was lower than in the open group by 48 hours following surgery.

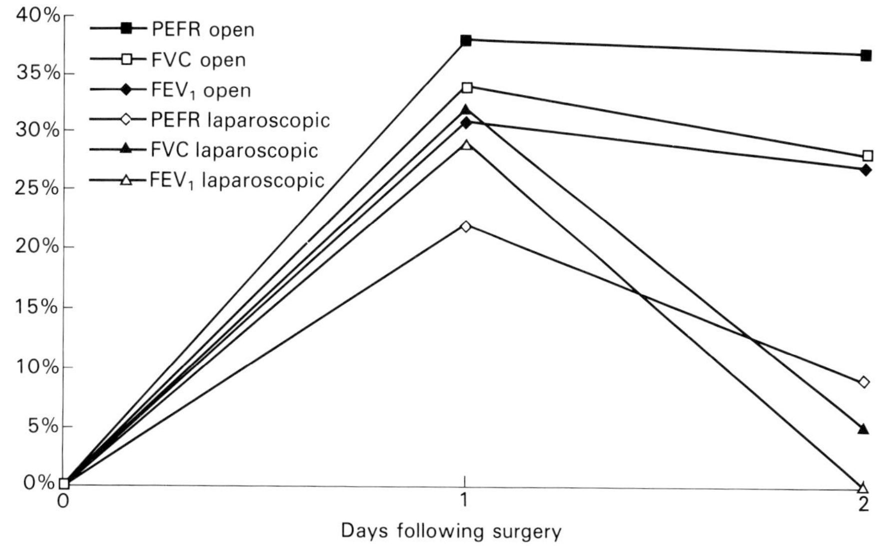

Fig. 7.3 Percentage reduction in lung function following nephrectomy. Postoperative pulmonary function as assessed by spirometry and peak-flowmetry were better preserved in the laparoscopic nephrectomy group.

than in the open group by 48 hours following surgery. Postoperative pulmonary function, as assessed by spirometry and peak-flowmetry, were better preserved in the laparoscopic group (Fig. 7.3). There was no significant difference between the two groups in respect of arterial blood gases, urinary noradrenalin or dopamine excretion.

The metabolic response to operative laparoscopy

It is interesting to speculate why there appears to be little metabolic advantage in performing a laparoscopic rather than an open cholecystectomy, whereas performing nephrectomy via a laparoscopic approach seems to elicit a significantly smaller stress response than by open operation. Access to the gallbladder by any of the standard open approaches requires much less tissue trauma than does open nephrectomy, which usually involves the division of a considerable bulk of muscle. It is perhaps not too surprising, therefore, that the metabolic consequences of performing the same operation using a minimal access approach are similar in the case of cholecystectomy but dissimilar in the case of nephrectomy. It appears that a laparoscopic approach to an operation in which the creation of access for its open counterpart involves substantial tissue trauma (such as nephrectomy) may be biologically superior. Conversely, the results also suggest that a minimal-access alternative to open procedures, such as minilap cholecystectomy and herniorrhaphy, in which the trauma of access is not dissimilar to that in the insertion of three or four trocars, cannot be justified on the grounds that it provokes a smaller stress response, unless it results in superior postoperative pulmonary function. The former operation fulfils these criteria, but the latter clearly does not.

Catecholamines

Two major pathways seem to be responsible for initiating and maintaining the stress response (Wilmore 1991): neural stimuli (which can be abolished by epidural anaesthesia (Brandt *et al.* 1978) and humoral factors (Table 7.1). It is interesting to note that the urinary VMA and adrenalin excretion was higher in the first 24 hours following laparoscopic cholecystectomy and nephrectomy, respectively, than in the open group. The cause may be increased afferent nerve impulse traffic to the pituitary–adrenal axis caused by stimulation of peritoneal stretch receptors by the pneumoperitoneum. The hypothesis is supported by the observation that the mean adrenalin excretion in the laparoscopic nephrectomy group during the second 24-hour period fell back to within the normal range (Fig. 7.2). A study of a further cohort of patients undergoing laparoscopic cholecystectomy, with half of the patients randomized to receive epidural anaesthesia and the other half not, is therefore indicated to further investigate this theory. In the case of the laparoscopic nephrectomy patients, an additional mechanism may be responsible for the findings: intraoperative adrenalin release by the adrenals during mobilization of the superior pole of the kidney, which is a difficult laparoscopic manoeuvre.

Cortisol

Horgan *et al.* (1992) have shown that laparoscopy is less immunotraumatic than open surgery by assessing spontaneous lymphocyte proliferation and responses to the mitogen phytohaemagglutinin in the cultured spleens of mice which had undergone laparotomy or laparoscopy. They also found higher mortality following infection with lipopolysaccharide in the laparoscopic group. These differences in immunity may be explained in part by the lower endogenous cortisol

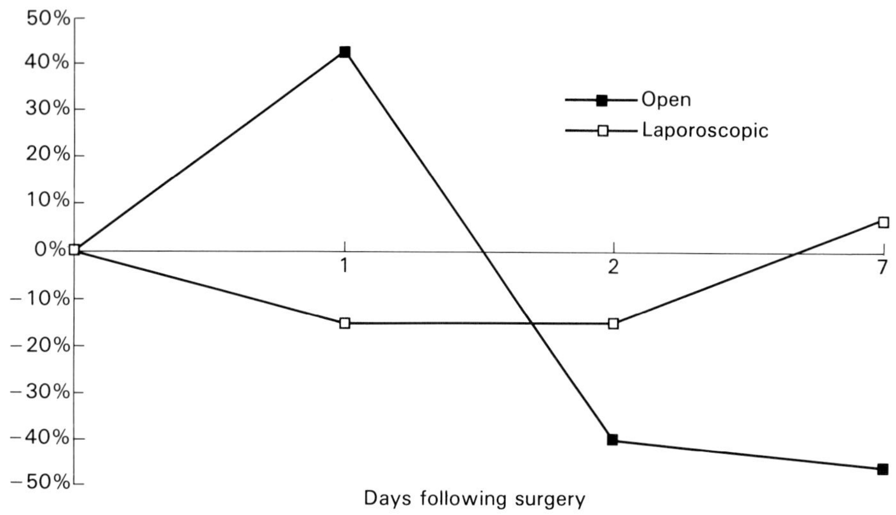

Fig. 7.4 Percentage change in 24-hour urinary urea excretion following both a laparoscopic and open nephrectomy. The differences are difficult to interpret, but it is likely that an improved post-operative hydration and reduced catabolism due to malignancy in the open nephrectomy group were responsible for the decline in the urea excretion seen in both groups.

secretion in the laparoscopic group, as noted in the authors' study. This has potential implications with regard to postoperative fluid retention, infection, wound-healing and, perhaps most importantly, recurrence following surgery for malignancy.

Nitrogen balance

The changes in perioperative urea excretion (Fig. 7.4) in the two nephrectomy groups are difficult to interpret. It seems likely that improved postoperative hydration and reduced catabolism due to malignancy were responsible for the decline in the urea excretion seen in the two groups. Assessment of the degree of catabolism by measurement of urinary urea excretion therefore seems to be inaccurate and further comment is inappropriate.

Calculation of nitrogen balance in patients whose hydration state is monitored by measurement of haematocrit and central venous pressure would give a better objective assessment of nitrogen flux, but one could still not control for errors due to the subclinical sepsis and malignant catabolism in many of the patients studied.

Generally, those patients who undergo minimal-access abdominal surgery have a much shorter, or absent, paralytic ileus, and they resume an oral diet sooner, than their conventionally operated counterparts. This constitutes an important difference between the two groups in the light of Windsor *et al.* (1988), who showed that recent food intake is more important than nutritional status for sound wound-healing.

Pulmonary function and pain perception

An upper abdominal wound typically results in a reduction of *FVC* and FEV_1 by 50% or more. These changes are caused by alteration of chest and abdominal wall dynamics and a decrease in lung volume due to basal atalectasis, respectively.

Diaphragmatic dysfunction following upper abdominal surgery is caused by splinting, due mainly to paralytic ileus, and paradoxical movement with respiration can occur. The pooled data from the three relevant studies confirms what common sense dictates, namely that the avoidance of a painful upper abdominal wound results in a lower postoperative analgesic requirement and better-preserved lung function. It also enables earlier postoperative patient mobilization and so reduces the likelihood of deep venous thrombosis and pulmonary embolism.

This has clear implications for patients with limited cardiorespiratory reserves. There can be no better example of this than the 101 kg patient in the laparoscopic nephrectomy series who had a mean reduction of only 19% in the three lung function parameters at 24 hours and 0% at 48 hours following operation. She would certainly have required thoracic epidural anaesthesia to allow acceptable gas exchange in the initial postoperative period had she undergone open surgery. The superior postoperative lung function should translate into a lower incidence of respiratory complications. Indeed, the only patient in the nephrectomy series who had a clinically apparent pulmonary complication (a hypoxic confusional state due to basal atalectasis) had undergone open nephrectomy.

The future

It is possible that the smaller stress response to laparoscopic nephrectomy results not only from less traumatic access, but also from gentler handling of tissues, and perhaps there is a lesson for us to learn here, which we can apply to our open surgical practice. Pharmacological and immune manipulation of the metabolic response to surgery may enable us to combine the excellent postoperative pulmonary function that follows operative laparoscopy with significantly decreased catabolism, fluid retention, muscle weakness, hyperglycaemia, and immunosupression, thus providing the ideal conditions for convalescence.

Nonsteroidal anti-inflammatory drugs have been shown (Wilmore, 1991) to reduce the effects of the cytokine interleukin-2, and studies are currently under way to investigate this effect in critically ill patients. Administration of monoclonal antibodies to other mediators of the stress response, such as tumour necrosis factor (Tracey *et al.* 1987), and platelet-activating factor (Sun & Hsueh 1988) also show great promise, as do insulin-like growth factor I (Guler *et al.* 1988) and epidermal growth factor (Brown *et al.* 1989), which have powerful anabolic properties.

Whatever the future of operative laparoscopy, it promises to be an exciting time for all those concerned with it. The greatest challenge that confronts us now is to devise laparoscopic operations that are both technically and biologically better that those attainable by today's open surgery.

References

Brandt M.R., Fernandes A., Mordhorst R. and Kehlet H. (1978) Epidural analgesia improves post-operative nitrogen balance. *British Medical Journal*, **1**, 1106–8.

Brown G.L., Nanney L.B., Griffen J. *et al.* (1989) Enhancement of wound healing by topical treatment with epidermal growth factor. *New England Journal of Medicine*, **321**, 76-9.

Chandra R.K. (1983) Nutrition, immunity and infection: present knowledge and future direction. *The Lancet*, **1**, 688–91.

Cuschieri A., Berci G., McSherry C.K. (1990) Laparoscopic cholecystectomy. *American Journal of Surgery*, **159**, 273.

Eden C.G. & Coptcoat M.J. (submitted for publication) The stress response to laparoscopic and open nephrectomy. *Journal of Minimally Invasive Therapy*.

Frazee R.C., Roberts J.W., Okeson G.C., *et al.* (1991) Open versus laparoscopic cholecystectomy. A comparison of postoperative pulmonary function. *Annals of Surgery*, **213**, 651–4.

Guler H.P., Zapf J., Froesch E.R. (1988) Recombinant human insulin-like growth factor I stimulates growth and has distinct effects on organ size in hypophysectomized rats. *Proceedings of the National Academy of Science of the USA*, **85**, 4889–93.

Horgan P.G., Fitzpatrick M., Couse N.F., Gorey T.F., Fitzpatrick J.M. (1992) Laparoscopy is less immunotraumatic than laparotomy. *Journal of Minimally Invasive Therapy*, **1**, 241–4.

Mealy K., Gallagher H., Barry M., Lennon F., Traynor O., Hyland J. (1992) Physiological and metabolic responses to open and laparoscopic cholecystectomy. *British Journal of Surgery*, **79**, 1061–4.

McMahon A.J., O'Dwyer P.J., Cruickshank A. *et al.* (1993) Metabolic changes after laparoscopic and minilap cholecystectomy: a randomised trial. Presentation at the annual meeting of the Surgical Research Society.

Platt M.P.W., Lovat P.E., Watson J.G., Aynsley-Green A. (1989) The effects of anaesthesia and surgery on lymphocyte populations and function in infants and children. *Journal of Pediatric Surgery*, **24**, 884–7.

Sun X.M. & Hsueh W. (1988) Bowel necrosis induced by tumour necrosis factor in rats is mediated by platelet-activating factor. *Journal of Clinical Investigations*, **81**, 1328–31.

Tracey K.J., Fong Y., Hesse D.G. *et al.* (1987) Anti-cachectin/TNF monoclonal antibodies prevent septic shock during lethal bacteraemia. *Nature*, **330**, 662–4.

Wilmore D.W. (1991) Catabolic illness. Strategies for enhancing recovery. *New England Journal of Medicine*, **325**, 695–702.

Windsor J.A., Knight G.S., Hill G.L. (1988) Wound healing response in surgical patients: recent food intake is more important than nutritional status. *British Journal of Surgery*, **75**, 135–7.

8: Laparoscopy for the Nonpalpable Testicle

M.J. COPTCOAT

Introduction

Laparoscopy acquired its first urological converts when it was realized that the nonpalpable testicle is best identified with laparoscopy, when often ultrasound or even computerized tomography is unhelpful (Weiss & Seashore 1987). Not only can the intra-abdominal testicle be found but, as is more common, the spermatic vessels can be followed down into the inguinal ring and this allows a subsequent accurate open exploration.

It was a logical step to utilize various operative laparoscopic techniques for biopsy or to remove such testicles (Thomas *et al.* 1992). A refinement in both instruments and techniques has allowed us to go one stage further and carry out a two-step orchidopexy with preliminary laparoscopic clip ligation of the spermatic vessels (Elder 1989, Bloom 1991).

Laparoscopic instrumentation

1 High-flow carbon dioxide insufflator
2 CCD camera and at least one monitor
3 Veress needle (safety)
4 0° 10mm laparoscope (300 optional)
5 Three 10mm ports with grips and converters/downsizers
6 Laparoscopic curved microscissors (diathermy connection)
7 Laparoscopic soft grasping forceps
8 Laparoscopic curved dissecting forceps
9 Endoclip* Applier (small/medium)

Technique

1 Under a general anaesthetic with muscle paralysis and assisted ventilation, the patient is put in a supine position with a 20–25° head-down tilt (Fig. 4.1a). A catheter is not usually required if the patient's bladder has recently emptied. Hip flexion is not required.

2 Formation of the pneumoperitoneum. The Veress needle is inserted at an angle of 45° into the empty pelvis (Fig. 4.2a). The position should be checked by aspiration and infusion of 5ml of saline, and during insufflation the intra-abdominal pressure should remain below

*A trademark of the United States Surgical Corporation (AutoSuture).

12 ml of mercury. In the hands of inexperienced laparoscopists, the disposable Veress needles with safety shield are safer. Previous major abdominal surgery is a relative contraindication. A previous appendicectomy is unlikely to have produced difficult intra-abdominal adhesions but anything more significant than this may produce an unnecessarily difficult procedure out of proportion to the open alternatives for the nonpalpable testicle.

3 Three 10 mm ports are placed according to the diagram (Fig. 8.1). The subumbilical port is for the telescope. The two secondary ports inserted along the lateral edges of the rectus sheath are for manipulative and dissecting instruments. The use of two 10 mm secondary ports allows the clip applicator to be introduced through either of these ports. The ports should be fixed with either grips or purse-string sutures.

4 The operator stands on the contralateral side of the patient whilst the camera-holder remains on the ipsilateral side.

5 The monitors should be at the bottom corners of the operating table (Fig. 8.2).

6 Adhesions to the sigmoid colon may need to be divided on the left-hand side before the testicular vessels become evident. The internal inguinal ring should be inspected first, because a small dysplastic testicle that has not been evident on CT or ultrasound may be sitting

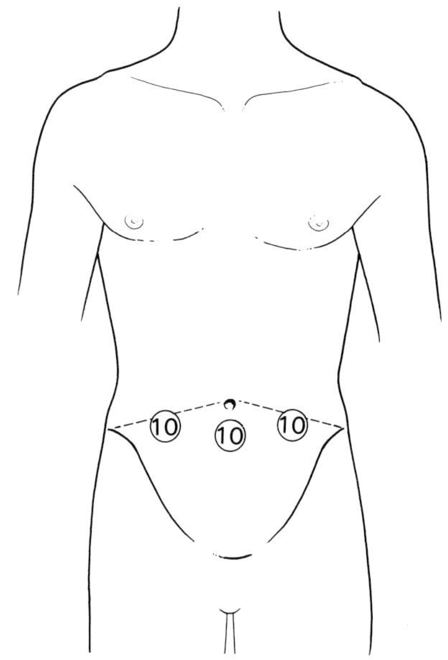

Fig. 8.1 The sites for the three 10 mm ports for a laparoscopic abdominal orchidectomy.

Fig. 8.2 The layout of equipment for a laparoscopic abdominal orchidectomy.

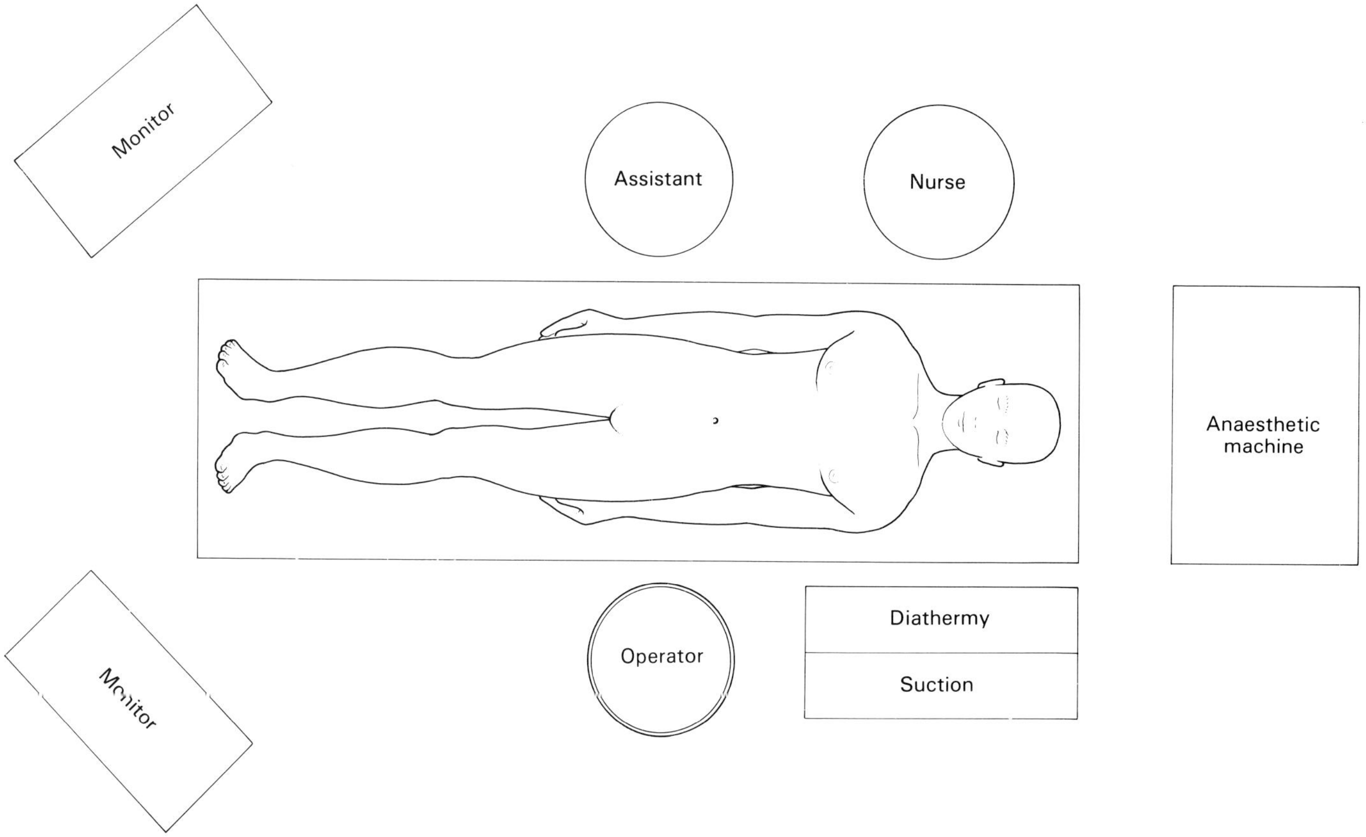

just inside the inguinal canal. The testicular vessels are a constant guide to the site of the testicle and it is only when they have been followed to their termination that one can conclude a complete absence when appropriate.

7 The patient's age and an assessment of the testicle's normality will determine the next step.

(a) If the testicle requires excision then the testicular vessels should be divided between pairs of clips (Fig. 8.3). The testicle can usually be drawn by forceps into the cannula of one of the ports and removed with the port at the end of the procedure. If the testicle is larger than 10 mm then the port incision will have to be enlarged and the testicle removed directly through this. Such operations require minimal dissection and haemostasis is only rarely a problem.

(b) The first stage of a Fowler–Stephens orchidopexy can be carried out laparoscopically. Once the intra-abdominal testicle has been identified and recognized as normal, a laparoscopic biopsy can be taken for frozen section if there is any doubt. The testicular artery and veins are divided between pairs of clips. Approximately six weeks after the first operation, the second but open stage of the orchidopexy can be carried out because the testicle will usually have retained an adequate blood supply from the artery to the vas.

8 The ports must be removed under direct vision. All carbon dioxide is evacuated.

9 To prevent wound-herniation, all wounds require a deep fascial suture. The skin can be sutured with a subcuticular absorbable suture or steristrips (Fig. 4.11); 3–5 ml of 0.5% marcaine are infiltrated into

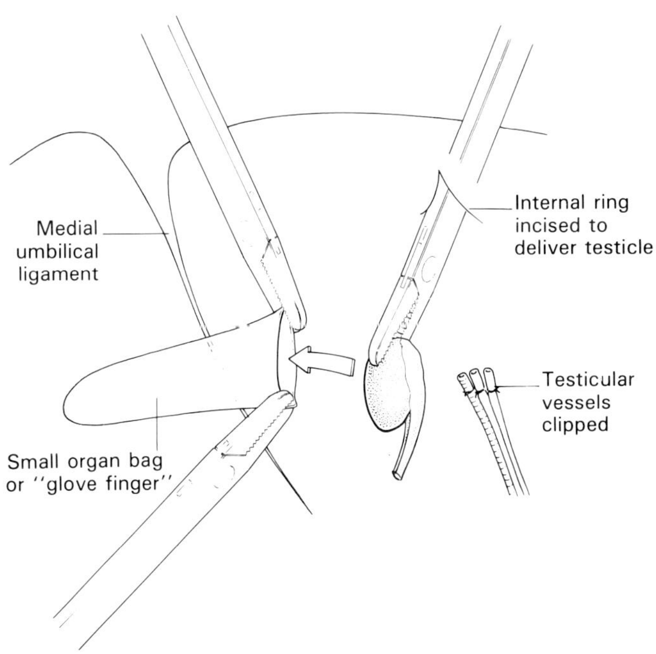

Fig 8.3 The testicular vessels to a dysplastic testicle just inside the internal inguinal ring have been clipped. The testicle is delivered into a small organ-retrieval bag or the finger from a large sterile surgical glove.

each wound. Patients require 1–2 hours hospitalization and can then be discharged home.

Discussion

Intra-abdominal cryptorchidism affects 8–9% of the cryptorchid population. It is generally accepted that these intra-abdominal testicles have a four-fold increased risk of malignancy compared to inguinal testicles and a 20–46-fold increased risk of malignancy compared to scrotal testicles. Additionally there is a significant increase in the number of germ-cell tumours encountered in unilateral cryptorchid testicles in patients who undergo orchidopexy after the age of 10. By the age of 10, the malignant potential of an intra-abdominal testicle outweighs the cosmetic benefit of orchidopexy. Prophylactic orchidectomy is appropriate therefore after this age and some have even suggested this protocol for children of more than six years of age. At whatever age orchidectomy is performed, the laparoscopic alternative is much less painful and results in a much more rapid return to normal activities.

Selective arteriography is an alternative diagnostic method for identifying an intra-abdominal testicle. It is less invasive than laparoscopy but carries the distinct disadvantage of being only a diagnostic tool: no further therapeutic action can be taken. Laparoscopy is slightly more invasive and requires a general anaesthetic but at least the testicle can either be excised or the spermatic vessels clipped to allow a second-stage orchidopexy.

References

Elder J.S. (1989) Laparoscopy and Fowler–Stephens orchidopexy in the management of the impalpable testis. *Urological Clinics of North America*, **16**: 2, 399–411.

Bloom D. (1991) Two-step orchiopexy with pelvioscopic clip ligation of spermatic vessels. *Journal of Urology*, **145**, 1030–3.

Thomas M.D., Mercer L.C., Saltzein E.C. (1992) Laparoscopic orchidectomy for unilateral intra-abdominal testis. *Journal of Urology*, **148**, 1251–3.

Weiss R.M. & Seashore J.H. (1987) Laparoscopy in the management of the nonpalpable testis. *Journal of Urology*, **138**, 344–82.

9: Laparoscopic Varicocelectomy

M.J. COPTCOAT AND A.D. JOYCE

Introduction

A varicocele is an abnormal tortuosity and dilatation of the testicular veins within the spermatic cord. A varicocele is found in approximately 15% of the general population and in at least 35% of infertile men (Greenberg 1977). It is also clear, however, that not all varicoceles are associated with abnormalities of the semen. Varicoceles do not occur with equal frequency on the left and right sides, as approximately 90% are left-sided.

Differences in the venous drainage patterns on the right and left testicular veins may account for this left-sided predominance. The left testicular vein drains into the left renal vein whereas the right testicular vein drains into the inferior vena cava.

In addition, there is a higher incidence of absent venous valves in the left side than in the right (Ahlberg *et al.* 1966). Unilateral right-sided varicoceles are uncommon. They raise the possibility of thrombosis or occlusion of the vena cava or situs inversus. Approximately 10% of patients present to infertility clinics with bilateral varicoceles, but the incidence may be much higher if epidemiological studies were repeated with doppler ultrasound rather than depending on the clinical findings alone.

Patients with a varicocele can present with testicular growth retardation in adolescence or as an adult with either subfertility or symptoms of a dragging discomfort in the scrotum. The latter presentation can be successfully managed by various methods of ligation or occlusion of the dilated testicular veins. It is unusual for any such procedure not to remove the symptoms even though there is a varied but high incidence of residual and recurrent varicocele.

One presumes that the venous congestion has at least been lowered below a threshold at which symptoms of discomfort are experienced. However, such a therapeutic strategy is not suitable for the patient with a varicocele who presents with subfertility. This group of patients deserve the procedure that completely abolishes the varicocele, has the least recurrence rate and is associated with improved male fertility.

Traditional approaches to the surgical repair of a varicocele include retroperitoneal (Palomo 1949) and inguinal (Ivanissevich 1960) operations. A hydrocele is a major complication of these operations. Szabo & Kessler (1984) reviewed the incidence of hydrocele formation after varicocelectomy and found rates varying from 3% to 39%, and in their own series an incidence of 7.2%. The protein concentration of the hydrocele fluid indicated that lymphatic obstruction was the cause of hydrocele formation after varicocelectomy.

Testicular atrophy is the most devastating complication of varicocelectomy, but it is rarely reported and its true incidence is unknown. Human studies suggest that ligation of the testicular artery is associated with a substantial risk of testicular injury during orchidopexy but this may only be relevant to those varicocele ligations within the inguinal canal. The high Palomo approach probably avoids this complication because testicular artery interruption takes place above the vas and its own arterial supply, which will act as a potential collateral source to the testicle. However, even a relative decrease in arterial flow may affect spermatogenesis without overt atrophy or morphological changes.

The incidence of persistent or recurrent varicocele following surgical repair in adults varies from 5% to 45% (Rothman *et al.* 1981, Belgrano *et al.* 1984) and appears to be even more common after repair of the paediatric varicocele. Venography of recurrent varicoceles has revealed that most recurrences are the result of midretroperitoneal or low inguinal parallel collaterals (Sayfan *et al.* 1981, Murray *et al.* 1986) but 7% of all recurrences appear to be due to scrotal collaterals (Kaufman *et al.* 1983).

Attempts at decreasing the complication rates following varicocelectomy have led to the development of microsurgical approaches which have the advantages of identification and preservation of the testicular artery and lymphatics and decrease the incidence of hydrocele formation and testicular artery injury. Intraoperative venography performed at the time of conventional varicocelectomy identifies the venous collaterals but markedly increases the operating time and still results in a significant incidence of varicocele recurrence similar to the disappointing results of percutaneous embolization (Kaufman *et al.* 1983, Porst *et al.* 1984).

Goldstein *et al.* (1992) have recently brought these issues into focus and has described a technique of open microsurgical (× 8 magnification) varicocelectomy with delivery of the testicle, division of gubernacular vessels, sparing of the testicular artery and lymphatics: 640 of these procedures were carried out in 429 men. Among 382 men available for follow-up examination from six months to seven years postoperatively, no hydroceles and no cases of testicular atrophy were found.

A total of four unilateral recurrent varicoceles (0.6%) was identified. Four scrotal haematomas occurred (0.6%) but no other complications. Preoperative and postoperative semen analyses were obtained in 271 men. They showed a statistically significant increase in sperm count, in motility and in normal forms. The pregnancy rate was 43% of couples followed for a minimum of six months postoperatively.

These results are vastly superior to previously reported alternative procedures and if reproducible by others should become the gold standard for varicocelectomy techniques.

The laparoscopic varicocelectomy is one of the most commonly performed laparoscopic procedures in urology departments but its clinical role has been much less clear than its use in exposing urologists to relatively straightforward operative laparoscopy. However, it has suffered from the early concept of trying to copy by laparoscopic means an established open procedure; in this case, the high Palomo testicular vein ligation. The most effective laparoscopic varicocelectomy technique must produce results similar to those reported by Goldstein and still have clear-cut advantages in minimizing the trauma of access and the delay in returning to normal activities.

The current laparoscopic telescopes and imaging systems have a potential magnification factor of up to three times. This has often been a disadvantage to the surgeon who is not used to having his or her nose right up against the object. But it should now be exploited as a form of internal operating microscope. In this respect it can be used to identify closely the testicular vessels beneath the peritoneum. Lymphatic and testicular artery ligation can be avoided whilst the spermatic vessels are left *in situ* free of tension because there is no need to bring them up to the surface. Such accurate dissection demands attention to the precise anatomy of the spermatic vessels (a recurrent theme in laparoscopy), where anatomical layers or linings are better appreciated and can be dissected more precisely than at open surgery.

Anatomy of the spermatic vessels

Beck *et al.* (1992), using an operating microscope with × 8 magnification have shown that the testicular veins and artery run within the internal spermatic fascia.

In 79 of 115 ligations (69%), a solitary testicular artery was identified. Two arteries were found in 27% and three arteries in 4% of men. In 50% of the 79 spermatic cords with a single testicular artery, the artery was adherent to the posterior surface of a large internal spermatic vein.

In 16 of the 31 cases in which two testicular arteries were identified, the artery was within two separate complexes of veins. Beck also describes an average of 3.6 (range 1–8) lymphatics within the internal spermatic fascia, a dilated vasal vein in 7% of cases and a dilated external spermatic vein separate from the spermatic cord and perforating the floor of the inguinal canal in 37% of cases.

Thus the laparoscopic varicocelectomy must be carried out in a meticulous way, avoiding the testicular arterial supply and, where possible, the lymphatics. The vas should be inspected for a dilated vasal vein and the peritoneum should be opened behind the inguinal canal to exclude a dilated external spermatic vein. The enclosing fascial sheaths require sharp, precise dissection which is best performed with fine scissors.

One cannot identify the gubernacular vessels during a laparoscopic varicocelectomy but their role is still unclear and should be left to provide venous drainage from the testicle through veins unaffected by the pathophysiological defect of a varicocele.

Instrumentation

1 High-flow carbon dioxide insufflator
2 CCD camera and at least one monitor
3 Veress needle (safety)
4 0° 10mm laparoscope (30° optional)
5 Three 10mm ports with grips and converters/downsizers
6 Laparoscopic curved microscissors (diathermy connection)
7 Laparoscopic soft grasping forceps
8 Laparoscopic curved dissecting forceps
9 Endoclip* Applier (small)

Technique

1 Under a general anaesthetic with muscle paralysis and assisted ventilation, the patient is put in a supine position with a 20–25° head-down tilt (Fig. 4.1a). A catheter is not usually required if the patient's bladder has recently emptied. Hip flexion is not required.
2 Formation of the pneumoperitoneum (Fig. 4.1): the Veress needle is inserted at an angle of 45° into the empty pelvis. The position should be checked by aspiration and infusion of 5ml of saline. The intra-abdominal pressure should remain below 12ml of mercury during insufflation. In the hands of inexperienced laparoscopists, the disposable Veress needles with a safety shield are safer. Previous major abdominal surgery is a relative contraindication. A previous appendicectomy is unlikely to have produced difficult intra-abdominal adhesions, but anything more significant than this may produce an unnecessarily difficult procedure out of proportion to the open alternatives that remain for a varicocelectomy. The Veress needle should be inserted through a subumbilical incision in an unscarred abdomen but in the presence of an appendicectomy scar, it is wise either to insert the Veress needle at the lateral edge of the left rectus sheath where one of the secondary ports would normally be placed, or to introduce the first port with a Hasson cut-down technique in this lateral position.

*A trademark of the United States Surgical Corporation (AutoSuture).

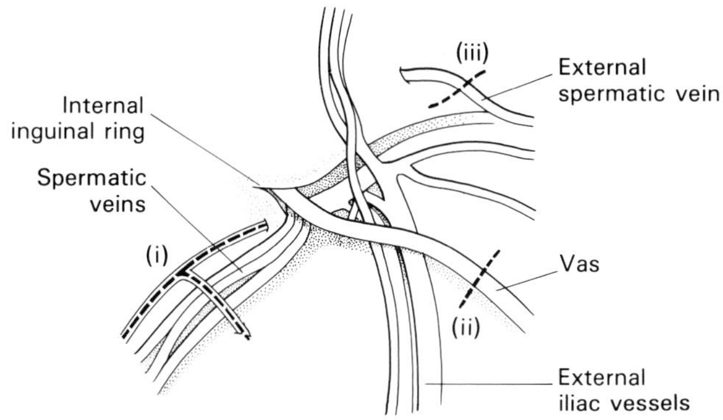

Fig. 9.1 The anatomy of the pelvic venous drainage from a varicocele, including (i) the internal spermatic veins, (ii) the vasal vein (iii) the external spermatic vein, and the peritoneal incisions required for a laparoscopic varicocelectomy.

3 Three 10mm ports are placed according to the diagram in Chapter 8 (Fig. 8.1). The subumbilical port is used for the telescope. A 30° telescope is sometimes useful if the sigmoid colon is full, because this allows visualization over the top and down onto the testicular vessels. The two secondary ports along the lateral edges of the rectus sheath are for manipulative and dissecting instruments. The use of two 10mm ports allows the clip applier to be introduced through either of them. The ports should be fixed with either grips or purse-string sutures.

4 The operator stands on the contralateral side of the patient whilst the camera-holder stands on the ipsilateral side.

5 The monitors should be at the bottom corners of the operating table.

6 Adhesions to the sigmoid colon may need to be divided on the left-hand side before the testicular vessels become evident. The vas should be easily identified leaving the internal inguinal ring and coursing medially and downwards. The site of spermatic vessel dissection must be well away from the vas. The peritoneum is picked up and incised longitudinally for 2cm just lateral to the testicular vessels. A 1cm incision perpendicular to this in the peritoneum over the vessels allows greater exposure (Fig. 9.1). The internal spermatic fascia then requires a separate longitudinal incision before the individual veins can be identified. Close attention is required to discriminate between veins and the fine accompanying lymphatics. A single or double artery will lie very close to one or two of the veins respectively, and dissection between them must be very careful. Care must be taken not to place too much tension on these vessels so that a testicular artery does not go into spasm and remains identifiable by virtue of its pulsation. The use of a laparoscopic doppler probe to identify the artery is an advantage. As each vein is identified, it should be divided between double small clips on each side. Watch the tips of the clip to prevent catching adjacent lymphatics or small nerves. Division of each vein in turn will allow closer inspection and more accurate dissection of the remaining contents of the internal spermatic fascia. Indiscriminate use of diathermy should be avoided to prevent inappropriate vessel ablation. A swab is preferable to irrigation and suction in these cases. The gauze swab should be connected to a nylon or silk retention suture via one of the ports. When all of the testicular veins have been divided, one's attention should turn to the vas. A small peritoneal incision is made over the vas and any possible dilated vasal vein obliterated with diathermy or a clip. Any possible external spermatic vein can only be seen if the peritoneum is incised directly behind the inguinal canal (Fig. 9.2). If such a vessel is present, it will arise from the medial aspects of the canal and so a small incision of just 1 cm in length at the medial end of the canal is sufficient to identify such a vein. If found, this can again be divided between clips.

Excellent haemostasis should be the norm. Any loose swabs should be withdrawn. If a bilateral varicocelectomy is required, the same ports can be used but we suggest that the operator and cameraman switch positions.

8 The ports must be removed under direct vision. All carbon dioxide is evacuated.

9 Wounds require a deep fascial suture to prevent wound-herniation. The skin can be either sutured with a subcuticular absorbable suture or steristrip. Patients require two to three hours to recover and can then be discharged home.

Complications

The laparoscopic varicocelectomy can be carried out as a day-case procedure. Only two of the patients in King's College Hospital have required an overnight stay and in both cases, this was for persistent nausea because of the use of inappropriate opiate analgesia peroperatively. Complications can otherwise be described as general to laparoscopy or specific to this procedure.

General complications

Veress needle or trocar injuries are extremely rare, probably due to the universal use of disposable equipment with safety shields. However, there are occasional reports of significant visceral and vascular injuries due to incorrect placement of the first port.

Perforation of the bifurcation of the aorta or iliac vessels is a very real but rare complication (less than 0.5%) and serves to remind us that the laparoscopic varicocelectomy must be shown to be a superior operation to its open counterparts which never carry such a catastrophic risk. Carbon dioxide absorption is not a problem because the procedure is usually over within 30–40 minutes.

In our series of 48 patients at King's College Hospital, there have been three cases of preperitoneal Veress needle malplacement and

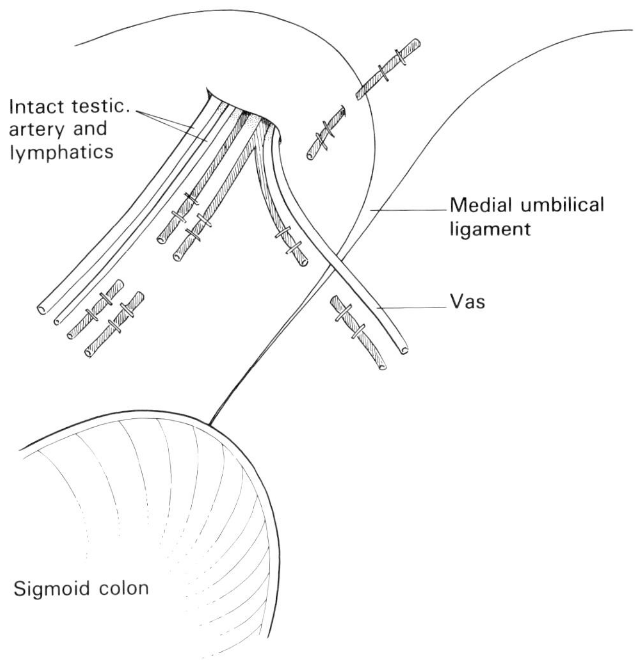

Fig. 9.2 The internal spermatic veins, sparing the lymphatics and the artery, together with the vasal and external spermatic veins, have been clipped and divided. Division is necessary to prevent recanalization. The veins rarely seem dilated in the head-down position. Inadvertent division of the testicular artery sometimes occurs, but this does not seem to have any serious clinical sequelae.

two superficial epigastric arterial incidents with the placement of secondary ports. Neither of these two types of complication have prevented a successful completion of the procedure and all occurred in the hands of relatively inexperienced staff.

Malpositioning of the Veress needle into the preperitoneal space can still sometimes produce a false-negative infusion and aspiration test. One should be alerted to this problem when the initial insufflation pressure rises immediately to 12mm of mercury or above. Early identification of this complication will allow the Veress needle to be placed into the peritoneum or, if necessary, at a distant site. The slow recognition of this complication leads to preperitoneal insufflation and it is thereafter more difficult to insert any of the ports and the patient is often uncomfortable postoperatively with superficial emphysema.

A superficial inferior epigastric artery rupture is usually only noticed upon removal of a port because the cannula has been tamponading the damaged artery. A clue to its damage sometimes comes from blood slowly trickling down the cannula inside the patient. If this is the case, a suture should be placed through the whole abdominal wall around the suspected site. This is best achieved by using a Stamey needle under direct intraperitoneal visualization. The suture can be threaded into the eye of the needle after two passes and the two ends brought onto the outside of the abdominal wall and tied. Quite large haematomas can form in the rectus sheath if this complication fails to be noticed, sometimes producing a drop in haemoglobin of 1–2g/dl.

Specific complications

There have been no specific complications in our series of patients at King's College Hospital. Aaberg *et al.* (1991), Hagood *et al.* (1992) and Donovan & Winfield (1992a, 1992b) have all reported a series where there is an absence of specific complications relating to the varicocelectomy, which reflects the ease of the technique and its safety once the ports have been inserted.

Donovan has felt that the risk, although small, of trocar injury has led him to utilize the open Hasson technique for the introduction of the first telescope port.

Discussion of results

Both Hagood *et al.* (1992) and Donovan & Winfield (1992a) have published results of their experience with the laparoscopic varicocelectomy. Hagood's series includes 10 patients with a mixture of clinical indications for a varicocelectomy. Four of these patients had bilateral varicocelectomies. There was no residual or recurrent varicocele demonstrated on either clinical or doppler examination in this series and complications were minimal. His technique was to identify the veins in as accurate a way as possible, and he was able to identify and leave the testicular artery preserved in each case. The procedure was particularly valuable for those patients with bilateral varicoceles because the same ports could be used. Donovan's series contained 14 patients. Five were bilateral. The clinical indications were all for oligospermia. Again, there were no recurrences in this series on follow-up, but this was based on clinical examination only. A return to normal activity was measured and there was found to be a mean of 3.4 days after the procedure. Several of the patients had undergone previous abdominal surgery and his recommendation is to introduce the first 10mm port by the open Hasson technique. The adhesions from an appendicectomy are rarely significant unless the patient gives a history of preceding peritonitis and this is not an absolute indication for the Hasson technique but may be preferred by the very cautious.

On the other hand, a more significant predictor of intra-abdominal adhesions such as a lower midline or paramedian incision should be a contraindication to a laparoscopic varicocelectomy. There seems little point in carefully dissecting these and both prolonging a simple operation and increasing the morbidity. An alternative open-groin approach would on balance be best in these cases.

One can, however, follow the logic of Donovan's later argument (Donovan & Winfield 1992b) where he recommends that all pelvic laparoscopy be initiated with the open introduction of the first port to avoid absolutely the rare vascular injuries caused sometimes by the

Veress needle, more often by the blind introduction of the first port a shielded trocar is not used. This debate will have to continue until the 'safety' ports have been evaluated over many years.

Donovan & Winfield (1992b) have also gone on to compare the use of the Nd:YAG laser for dissection and coagulation and have found this to be superior to using scissors and diathermy but if this is a rerun of the laparoscopic cholecystectomy–laser study then the minimal benefits will be overridden by the extra costs and frustration of wearing protective eyewear.

In our own series at King's College Hospital, we have seen the evolution of a new procedure that reflects the advantages that a laparoscopic technique brings. Our first 15 patients underwent mass ligation of the spermatic veins. The testicular artery was not identified in six cases although there were no unwanted sequelae of testicular pain or subsequent atrophy. The second series of 15 patients underwent a slightly more sophisticated laparoscopic procedure where the veins were identified, clipped and divided behind the retroperitoneum, the peritoneum was opened behind the inguinal canal and any external spermatic vein (three cases) if present was also clipped and any dilated vasal veins were also similarly dealt with (two cases). This was, to all intents and purposes, a much more complete and radical ablation of the venous drainage of the testicle. In this group of patients, there were no recurrences on either clinical or doppler follow-up after six months which is in contrast to four recurrent varicoceles in our first series (27%). The disadvantage of the more complete venous ablation was the formation of lymphatic hydroceles in three cases (20%).

In order to avoid this complication and yet still achieve the same high standard of success for the varicocelectomy, we have concentrated on using the laparoscope as an endoscopic operating microscope. In our most recent series of 10 cases, the same degree of venous ablation has been achieved but at the same time, the cord has been much more carefully dissected with finer instruments and small clips have been used. The testicular artery and associated lymphatics have all been identified and left intact. This has produced the ideal result of complete success in eradicating the varicocele and we have also avoided the complication of a lymphatic hydrocele. This seems to be a good example of how a laparoscopic procedure should not merely be a copy of a previously described open counterpart. However, we will not see the additional benefits of using the laparoscope as an endoscopic operating microscope until the telescopes themselves have further increased magnification and the instrumentation becomes more refined for delicate dissection. The length of the operation in all surgeons' hands has become dramatically shorter with experience, and no more than 30–40 minutes should be needed for a unilateral varicocelectomy.

The advantage as stated above of a bilateral varicocelectomy carried out through the same ports means that this only adds a mere 10–15 minutes on to the procedure if this is indicated. The cost of using disposable equipment throughout the procedure has been criticized in the past, and where we have to compete in terms of health economics with other simple day-case alternatives, the use only of a nondisposable first telescope port and disposable sharp microscissors seems indicated now.

The future of the laparoscopic varicocelectomy is much more secure because it has now evolved into a refined technique that matches the gold standard set by Goldstein *et al.* (1992) but at the same time reduces the trauma of access and so allows the patient to return to normal activities much quicker than even the most minor open alternative.

References

Aaberg R.A., Vancaille T.G., Schuessler W.W. (1991) Laparoscopic varicocele ligation: A new technique. *Fertility and Sterility*, **56**, 776.

Ahlberg N.E., Bartley O., Chidekel N. (1966) Right and left gonadal veins: An anatomical and statistical study. *Acta Radiologica*, **4**, 593.

Beck E.M., Schlegel P.N., Goldstein M. (1992) Intraoperative varicocele anatomy: A macroscopic and microscopic study. *Journal of Urology*, **148**, 1190–4.

Belgrano E., Puppo P., Quattrini S., Trombetta C., Giuliani L. (1984) The role of venography and sclerotherapy in the management of varicocele. *European Urology*, **10**, 124.

Donovan J.F., Winfield H.N. (1992a) Laparoscopic varix ligation. *Journal of Urology*, **147**, 77.

Donovan J.F., Winfield H.N. (1992b) Laparoscopic varix ligation with the Nd:YAG laser. *Journal of Endourology*, **6**: 2, 165–71.

Goldstein M., Gilbert B., Dicker A.P., Dwosk J., Gnecco C. (1992) Microsurgical inguinal varicocoelectomy with delivery of the testis: An artery and lymphatic sparing technique. *Journal of Urology*, **148**, 1808–11.

Greenberg S.H. (1977) Varicocele and male fertility. *Fertility and Sterility*, **28**, 699.

Hagood P.G., Mehan D.J., Wrischeck J.H., Andrus C.H., Parra R.O. (1992) Laparoscopic varicocelectomy: Preliminary report of a new technique. *Journal of Urology*, **147**, 73.

Ivanissevich O. (1960) Left varicocele due to reflux: Experience with 4,470 operative cases in forty-two years: *Journal of the International College of Surgeons*, **34**, 742.

Kaufman S.L., Kadir S., Barth K.H., Smyth J.W., Walsh P.C., White R.I. Jr (1983) Mechanisms of recurrent varicocele after balloon occlusion or surgical ligation of the internal spermatic vein. *Radiology*, **147**, 435.

Murray R.R. Jr, Mitchell S.E., Kadir S. *et al.* (1986) Comparison of recurrent varicocele anatomy following surgery and percutaneous balloon occlusion. *Journal of Urology*, **135**, 286.

Palomo A. (1949) Radical cure of varicocele by a new technique: Preliminary report. *Journal of Urology*, **61**, 604.

Porst H., Bähren W., Lenz M., Altwein J.E. (1984) Percutaneous sclerotherapy of varicoceles—an alternative to conventional surgical methods. *British Journal of Urology*, **56**, 73.

Rothman C.M., Newmark H. III, Karson R.A. (1981) The recurrent varicocele—a poorly recognised problem. *Fertility and Sterility*, **35**, 552.

Sayfan J., Adam Y.G., Soffer Y. (1981) A natural 'venous bypass' causing post-operative recurrence of a varicocele. *Journal of Andrology*, **2**, 108.

Szabo R., Kessler R. (1984) Hydrocoele following internal spermatic vein ligation: A retrospective study and review of the literature. *Journal of Urology*, **132**, 924.

10: Laparoscopic Herniorraphy

M.J. COPTCOAT AND A.D. JOYCE

Introduction

Transabdominal repair of an inguinal hernia is not a new concept and many surgeons will readily perform such a procedure if associated with a concomitant laparotomy (La Roque 1932, Ger 1982, Marcy 1987). The laparoscopic approach to hernia repair is a natural progression from this concept. It has the advantage of avoiding a muscle-cutting incision and so postoperative pain is minimal. A tension-free prosthesis is fixed to the preperitoneal surface with metal clips to accomplish closure of the internal inguinal ring and to strengthen the weak posterior inguinal wall. This is similar to the open technique described by Nyhus *et al.* (1988). This laparoscopic placement could conceivably be the same for direct, indirect or even femoral hernias. There are very few large series of laparoscopic hernia repairs and certainly no long-term results are available as yet, but short-term results are very encouraging (Popp 1990).

The technique involves incising the peritoneum medially and laterally from the internal ring with point diathermy or scissors around the medial edge of the internal ring. The sac is then dissected free and either left open or closed (Ger *et al.* 1990) with an endoloop. A mesh plug can be introduced into the indirect hernial defect or a posterior wall herniorrhaphy can be undertaken by stapling a second mesh.

Laparoscopic instrumentation

1 High-flow carbon dioxide insufflator
2 CCD camera and at least one monitor
3 Veress needle (safety)
4 0° 10mm laparoscope (30° optional)
5 One 10mm port plus two 12mm ports with grips and converters/downsizers
6 Laparoscopic curved microscissors (diathermy connection)
7 Laparoscopic soft grasping forceps
8 Laparoscopic curved dissecting forceps
9 Laparoscopic hernia stapler
10 Nonabsorbable polypropylene mesh

Technique

1 Under a general anaesthetic with muscle paralysis and assisted

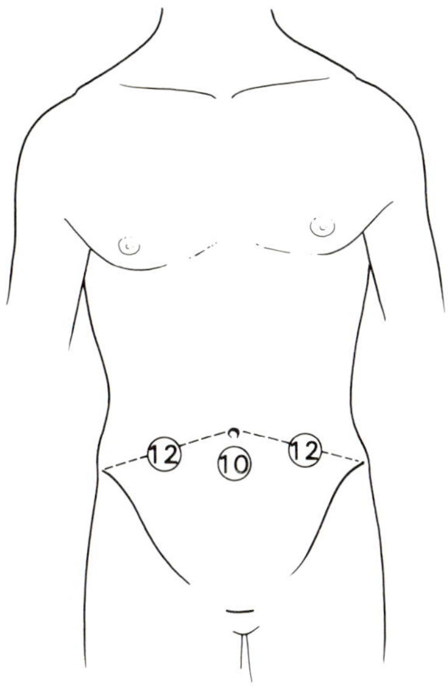

Fig. 10.1 Sites of the 10mm telescope port and two 12mm ports for manipulative and dissecting instruments in a laparoscopic inguinal herniorraphy.

ventilation, the patient is put in a supine position with a 20–25° head-down tilt (Fig. 4.1a). A catheter is not usually required if the patient's bladder has recently emptied. Hip flexion is not required.

2 Formation of the pneumoperitoneum (Fig. 4.1): the Veress needle is inserted at an angle of 45° into the empty pelvis. The position should be checked for aspiration by infusion of 5ml of saline and the intra-abdominal pressure should remain below 12ml of mercury during insufflation. In the hands of inexperienced laparoscopists, the disposable Veress needles with a safety shield are safer. Previous major abdominal surgery is a relative contraindication. A previous appendicectomy is unlikely to have produced difficult intra-abdominal adhesions, but anything more significant than this may produce an unnecessarily difficult procedure out of proportion to the open alternatives for a herniorrhaphy.

3 A 10mm port for the telescope is placed just below the umbilicus. Two 12mm ports are inserted along the lateral edges of the rectus sheath and these are for manipulative and dissecting instruments (Fig. 10.1). The use of two 12mm ports allows the sta,pling device to be inserted from either side which sometimes facilitates easier access to certain parts of the herniorrhaphy. The ports should be fixed either with grips or purse-string sutures.

4 The operator stands on the contralateral side of the patient whilst the camera holder stands on the ipsilateral side (Fig. 8.1).

5 The monitors should be at the bottom corners of the operating table.

6 Adhesions to the sigmoid colon may need to be divided on the left-hand side. An indirect hernial sac should be circumcised at the internal inguinal ring after the contents have been withdrawn back into the abdomen. The terminal portion is left free.

7 The peritoneum is then incised behind the back wall of the inguinal canal with scissors. The inferior epigastric vessels sometimes require division between clips if it looks as if they will prevent precise placement of the mesh. The peritoneum is dissected to reveal

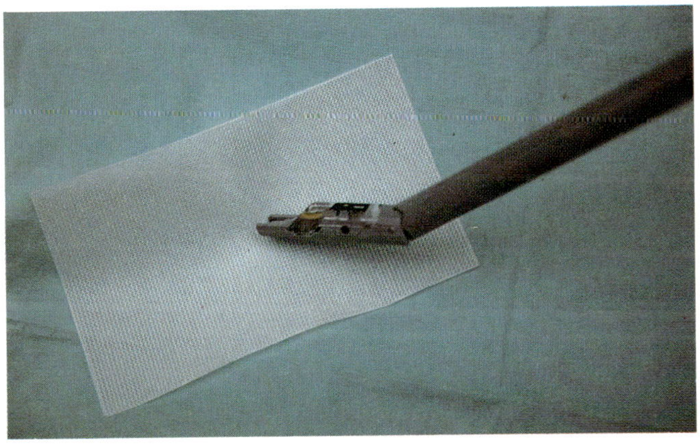

Fig. 10.2 A herniorraphy stapler that can be angled to produce a better contact.

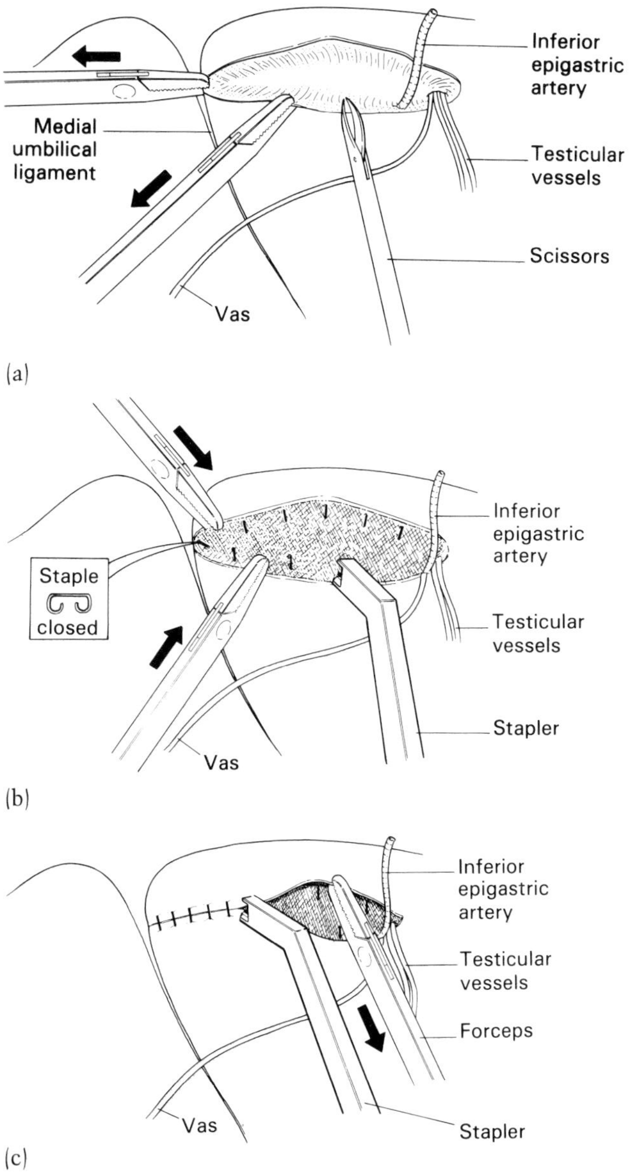

Fig. 10.3 (a) The peritoneum is dissected to reveal enough space for a mesh plug behind the weak posterior wall of the inguinal canal. (b) The tailored piece of mesh is stapled to the inguinal ligament below the conjoint tendon. (c) The peritoneum is brought back and stapled to cover the mesh.

enough space for the mesh (Fig. 10.3a). An approximate template can be measured using the known length of the forceps or scissors. The required size of mesh is then inserted and placed up against the back wall of the inguinal canal. It is stapled to the inguinal ligament below, the pubic tubercle medially and internal oblique aponeurosis superiorly (Fig. 10.3b). The stapler can be angulated to fire the staples perpendicular to the structures and if this is not possible, introduction of the stapler through the opposite side usually helps. The peritoneum is then brought back over to cover the mesh and can be either closed with a continuous suture or with further staples (Fig. 10.3c) The latter is much simpler and quicker. A direct hernia does not obviously require any dissection of a sac and the defect in the posterior wall of the inguinal canal can be enhanced by asking an assistant to place two or three fingers externally into the defect and dissection can take place around them. Otherwise the technique for herniorrhaphy is indentical to that of an indirect hernia.

8 The ports must be removed under direct vision. All carbon dioxide is evacuated.

9 All wounds require a deep fascial suture to prevent wound-hernias. The skin can be either sutured with a subcuticular absorbable suture or steristrip. Patients require two or three hours to recover and can then be discharged home. Patients should refrain from lifting more than a briefcase for three weeks.

Discussion

There is no doubt that currently available stapling instrumentation makes the laparoscopic herniorrhaphy a simple and straightforward procedure. However, its long-term results are unknown but earlier results are very encouraging and point to a recurrence rate that is at least as low as with an open herniorrhaphy (Corbitt 1991, Nolen *et al.* 1992). Unfortunately, the present stapling devices are quite expensive and it is difficult to rationalize this procedure against a day-case open herniorrhaphy, especially when done under local anaesthesia.

When a laparoscopic alternative drastically changes the morbidity and hospital stay, the increase in operating time and equipment is irrelevant, but in the case of a herniorrhaphy, this contrast is not apparent. The patients definitely experience far less postoperative discomfort following a laparoscopic herniorrhaphy and this is enough to keep most of us open-minded. The answer probably lies in nondisposable instrumentation being developed that will reduce the operating costs.

Discussion still takes place regarding the indirect sac and many surgeons are beginning to leave the sac free after excision and pack the inguinal canal with a Marlex mesh folded into a fan configuration. This is becoming the method of choice for treating indirect hernias whilst the stapling of a simple mesh over the posterior wall will probably be the best solution for direct inguinal hernias. Further follow-up is required to confirm these speculative thoughts.

References

Corbitt, J.D. (1991) Laparoscopic herniorrhaphy. *Surgical Laparoscopy and Endoscopy*, **1**, 23–25.

Ger R. (1982) The management of certain abdominal hernias by intra-abdominal closure of the neck. *Annals of the Royal College of Surgeons of England*, **64**, 342–4.

Ger R, Monroe K, Duvivier R *et al*: (1990) Management of indirect inguinal hernias by laparoscopic closure of the neck of the sac. *American Journal of Surgery*, **159**, 370–2.

LaRoque G.P. (1932) The intra-abdominal method of removing inguinal and femoral herniae. *Archives of Surgery*, **24**, 189–203.

Marcy H.O. (1987) The cure of hernia. *Journal of the American Medical Association*, **8**, 589–92.

Nolen M., Melichar R., Jennings W.C., McGee J. (1992) Use of a Marlex fan in the repair of direct and indirect hernias by laparoscopy. *Journal of Laparoendoscopic Surgery*, **2**, (2), 1061–4.

Nyhus L.M., Pollak R., Bombeck T.C., Conahue P.E. (1988) The preperitoneal approach and prosthetic buttress repair for recurrent hernia. *Annals of Surgery*, **208**, 733–7.

Popp L.W. (1990) Endoscopic patch repair of inguinal hernia in a female patient. *Surgical Endoscopy*, **4**, 10-12.

11: Laparoscopic Appendicectomy

M.J. COPTCOAT AND A.D. JOYCE

Introduction

In 1983, Professor Semm from Kiel (going under the label of a gynaecologist but truly a founding father of the minimally invasive surgical movement) reported the first case of an appendix removed solely with laparoscopic methods. At this time, it was not recommended that the procedure be applied to acute inflammation of the appendix and it was not until 1987 (Gangal & Gangal 1987) that the first report of laparoscopic surgery for acute appendicitis was published. Semm now has a vast experience of this technique and feels that the only contraindication is advanced gangrenous appendicitis (Semm 1991).

As an end organ, the appendix lends itself to easy removal by the laparoscope, although dissection is required if it is retrocaecal in situation. The blood supply of the appendix must be controlled and divided. The attachment to the caecum must be controlled to prevent any leakage of faecal material, but inversion of the stump is not required (Engstrom & Fenyo 1985). Because of the slightly larger fascial opening, the Hasson technique, using a larger cannula, permits the removal of an oedematous inflamed appendix.

Instrumentation

1 High-flow carbon dioxide insufflator
2 CCD camera and at least one monitor
3 Veress needle (safety)
4 0° 10mm laparoscope (30° optional)
5 One 10mm port, one 12mm port and two 5mm port, all with grips and converters/downsizers
6 Laparoscopic curved microscissors (diathermy connection)
7 Laparoscopic soft grasping forceps
8 Laparoscopic curved dissecting forceps
9 Laparoscopic forceps
10 Endoclip* Applier (medium/large)
11 Endo GIA* 30 stapler (optional)

Technique

1 Under a general anaesthetic with muscle paralysis and assisted

*A trademark of the United States Surgical Corporation (AutoSuture).

ventilation, the patient is put in a supine position with a 20–25° head-down tilt. A catheter is not usually required if the patient's bladder has recently emptied. Hip flexion is not required.

2 Formation of the pneumoperitoneum: the Veress needle is inserted at an angle of 45° into the empty pelvis. The position should be checked for aspiration by infusion of 5 ml of saline and the intra-abdominal pressure should remain below 12 ml of mercury during insufflation.

In the hands of inexperienced laparoscopists, the disposable Veress needles with a safety shield are safer. Previous major abdominal surgery is a relative contraindication because it may have produced difficult intra-abdominal adhesions, and this may produce an unnecessarily difficult procedure out of proportion to the open alternatives for an appendicectomy.

3 The ports are placed according to the diagram (Fig. 11.1). A subumbilical port is used for the telescope. The 12 mm port on the lateral edge of the left rectus sheath is for the optional Endo GIA 30 stapler if the appendix or mesoappendix prove to be difficult to dissect. The low midline 5 mm port 3–4 cm above the symphysis pubis is only necessary if extra retraction is required.

4 The operator stands on the contralateral side of the patient whilst the camera-holder stands on the ipsilateral side (Fig. 11.2).

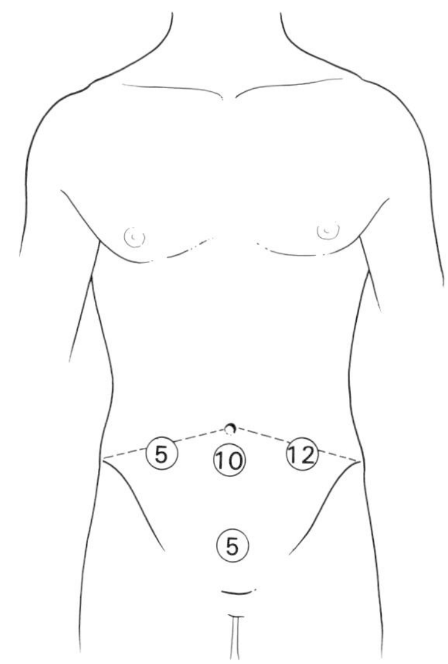

Fig. 11.1 The ports sites—two 5mm, one 10mm and one 12mm—for a laparoscopic appendicectomy.

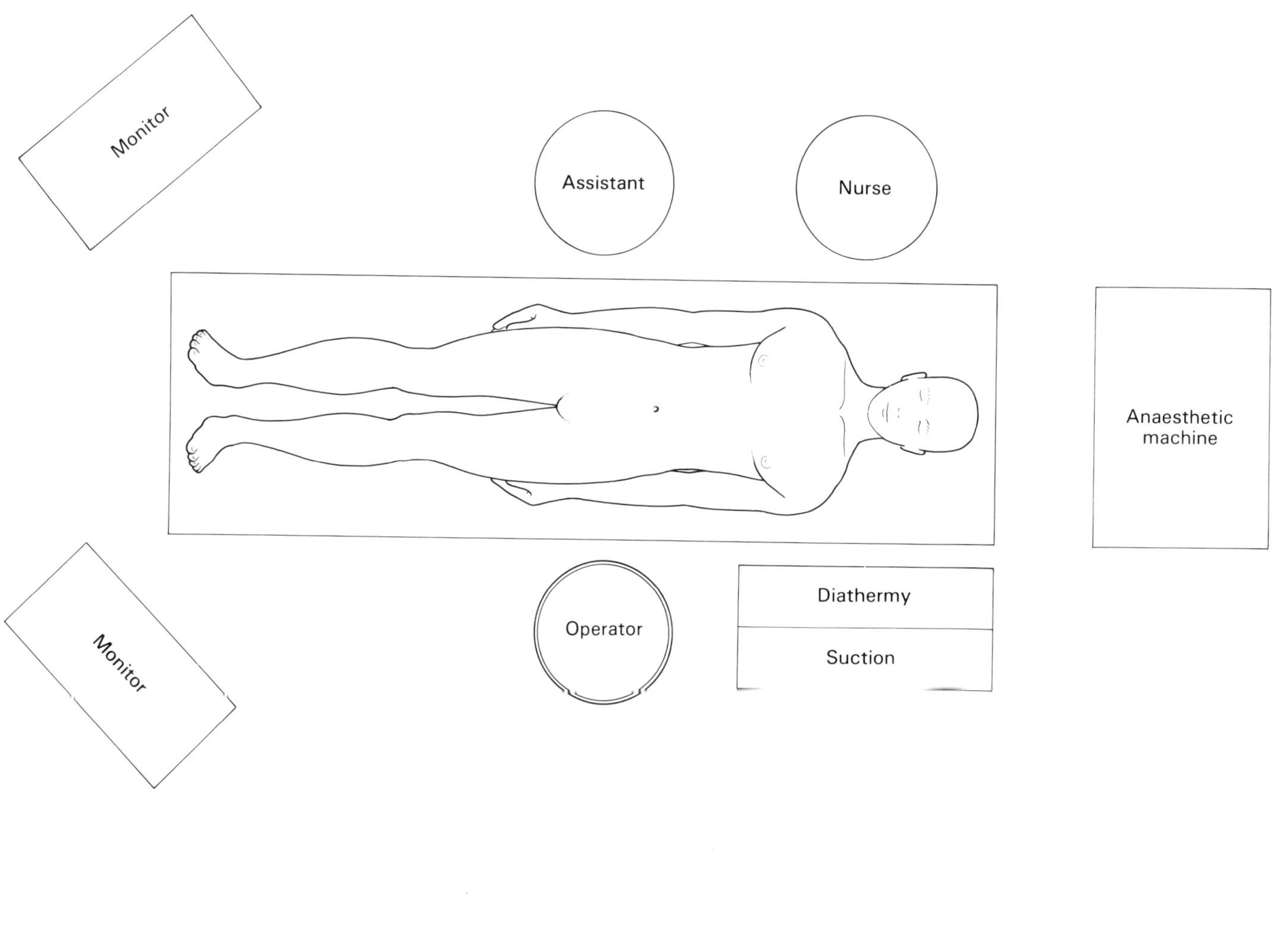

Fig. 11.2 The layout of equipment for a laparoscopic appendicectomy.

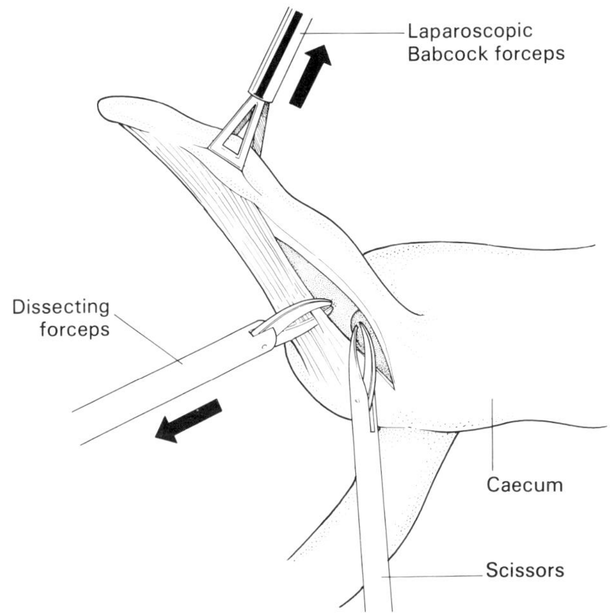

Fig. 11.3 The appendix is grasped with Babcock forceps and a window is made in the mesoappendix close to the base.

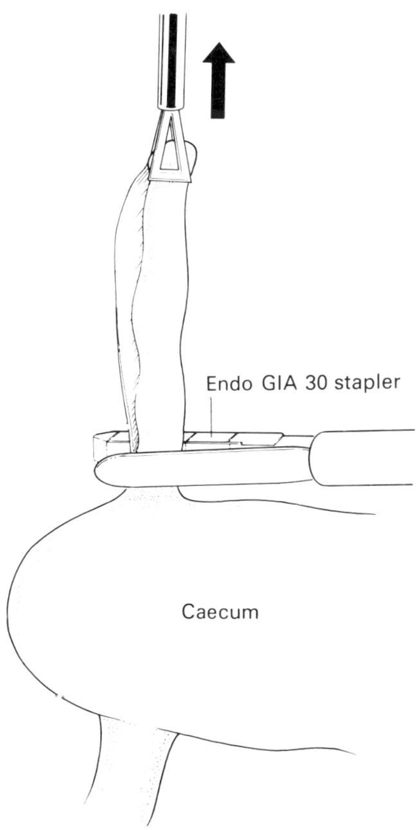

Fig. 11.4 The Endo GIA 30 stapler is used for both the mesoappendix and the appendix. It is important to measure the depth of the staples needed with a gauge before resecting the appendix.

5 The video monitors should be at the bottom corners of the operating table.

6 The appendix is grasped with soft forceps through the midline port. Dissection of adhesions is carried out with scissors and dissecting forceps through the lateral ports. A window is made in the mesoappendix close to the base of the appendix (Fig. 11.3).

If the mesoappendix is thick, then the safest method for haemostasis and division is to use the Endo GIA 30 stapler. Smaller vessels can be divided between double surgical clips. Ligatures can be used but each ligature requires extracorporeal knot formation and is generally quite time-consuming. The base of the freed appendix is crushed with forceps.

Again, the Endo GIA 30 stapler is very useful for a large appendix (Fig. 11.4) but a prepared endoloop made of either catgut or vicryl or Polysorb suture is sometimes appropriate. The appendix can usually be withdrawn through the 12 mm port. Take care to depress the flap valve or trumpet valve as the appendix is pulled through. The base of the appendix can be left, but it is usually our practice to bury this beneath a simple crisscross suture (Fig. 11.5) with the knot tied intracorporcally.

7 Excellent haemostasis should be the norm. Loose swabs should be withdrawn.

8 The ports must be removed under direct vision. All carbon dioxide is evacuated.

9 To prevent wound-herniation, all wounds require a deep fascial suture. The skin can be sutured with a subcuticular absorbable suture or steristripped. Patients can usually be discharged home on the following day.

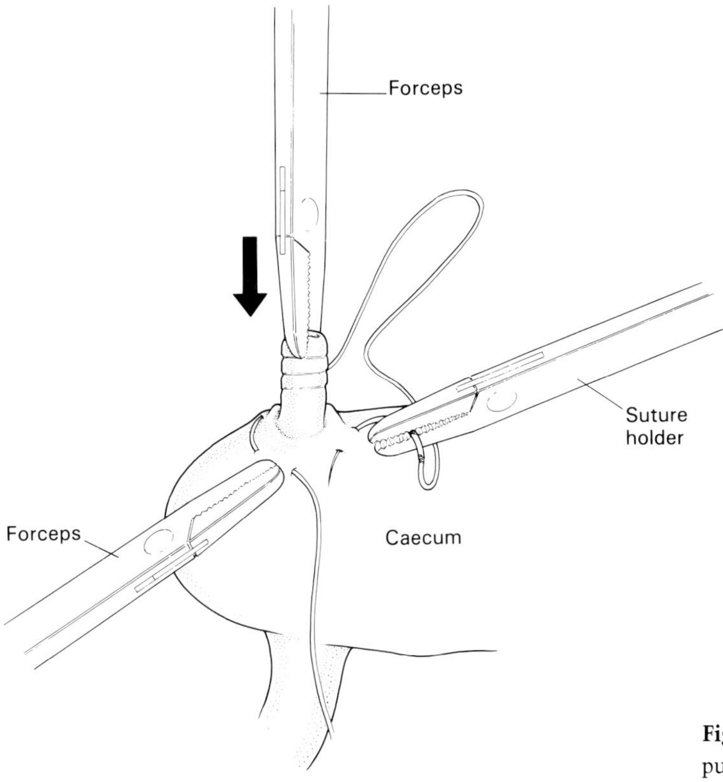

Fig. 11.5 The base of the appendix can be buried with either a purse-string or a simple crisscross suture.

Discussion

Because of the use of laparoscopy in making a diagnosis of right iliac fossa pain, it should now be unnecessary to remove a normal appendix. The introduction of diagnostic laparoscopy in this case alone will have obvious implications in terms of lower morbidity and better health economics.

Unfortunately, there are still many hospitals where a request for laparoscopic equipment by the emergency surgeon is greeted with groans and dismay by the operating theatre staff who have always been used to a very rapid open appendicectomy. Fortunately, this situation is now changing for the better. It seems a natural step to introduce secondary ports and carry out the appendicectomy with laparoscopic instrumentation. Even though it will take three or four times longer than its open counterpart, the benefits are enormous to the patient.

However, it is interesting to notice that whilst a simple laparoscopic appendicectomy for early appendicitis goes home the following day, a laparoscopic appendicectomy for quite advanced appendicitis still requires four or five days of hospitalization. This again points to the fact that, although laparoscopy minimizes the trauma of access, if we only copy the open operation once we are inside, any morbidity associated with internal dissection will still be seen following laparoscopic surgery.

References

Engstrom L & Fenyo G. (1985) Appendicectomy: An assessment of stump invagination. A prospective trial. *British Journal of Surgery*, **72**, 971–2.

Gangal I.I.T. & Gangal M.H. (1987) Laparoscopic appendectomy. *Endoscopy*, **19**, 127–9.

Schreiber J. (1987) Early experience with laparoscopic appendectomy in women. *Surgical Endoscopy*, **1**, 211–16.

Semm K. (1991) Endoscopic appendectomy. *Endoscopy*, **15**, 59–64.

12: Laparoscopic Pelvic Lymphadenectomy

M.J. COPTCOAT AND A.D. JOYCE

Introduction

The laparoscopic pelvic lymphadenectomy has become an established procedure in many urological and gynaecological departments for the staging of early carcinoma of the prostate, bladder, uterus and cervix (Gershman *et al.* 1990, Winfield *et al.* 1992, Schuessler *et al.* 1991, Parra *et al.* 1992, Coptcoat & Wickham 1992). For many, it has replaced an open pelvic lymphadenectomy, and in some centres its relatively low morbidity and high sensitivity and specificity have led surgeons to begin staging their pelvic cancer patients by way of a lymphadenectomy for the first time.

There is no doubt that the laparoscopic pelvic lymphadenectomy is both a reasonable and feasible procedure but this does not justify its use unless the finding of micrometastases in regional lymph nodes alters the management of a particular case. The answer varies slightly with each type of pelvic cancer and, more importantly, it varies with each individual patient. In general terms, one can say that surgical staging of lymph nodes is an attractive alternative to clinical non-invasive staging in the planning of therapy in the event of micrometastases in regional lymph nodes, because it is more accurate and provides precise histological documentation of disease extent, and it permits individualization of therapy on the basis of specific patterns of disease spread.

Various diagnostic modalities have been employed as alternatives to surgical exploration—for example, lymphangiography, computed tomography (CT) and magnetic resonance imaging (MRI). All are limited in their ability to delineate disease extent and they cannot compare with the accuracy of surgical staging (Loening *et al.* 1977, Benson *et al.* 1981, Feigen *et al.* 1987, Rifkin *et al.* 1990). This preliminary thesis should apply only if the combined morbidity and mortality of a laparoscopic exploration and definitive therapy do not outweigh the benefits accrued by the precise definition of disease.

A wider acceptance of a laparoscopic pelvic lymphadenectomy may directly benefit many patients who were referred for radiotherapy. In the past, surgeons and radiation oncologists have been hesitant strongly to encourage an open pelvic lymphadenectomy for patients who undergo external or interstitial radiotherapy (Ray *et al.* 1976). The problem with this philosophy has been that many patients will have been understaged and will therefore receive therapy, with its attendant side effects, inappropriately and without being cured.

Radiation oncologists will often argue that their 5-, 10- and 15-year actuarial results are comparable to those of most surgical series for all pelvic cancers, despite the fact that radiotherapy patients were not pathologically staged or were not technically or medically fit for surgery (Bagshaw *et al.* 1987).

This is a contentious statement, and many surgeons would point to so-called definitive papers which show that surgery is superior (Paulson *et al.* 1982).

Whatever the specific argument in each type of cancer, there is every reason to believe that the introduction of a laparoscopic staging pelvic lymphadenectomy for patients referred for radiotherapy would lead to better patient selection and ultimately improve the stated results in radiotherapy reports.

A laparoscopic pelvic lymphadenectomy is an accurate staging procedure only and is in no way therapeutic. It cannot be seen as a complete clearance of all relevant nodes in all patients and so cannot fit in to the management protocol of patients where radical surgery and a radical lymphadenectomy is pursued in the presence of positive lymph nodes, as suggested by Zincke *et al.* (1981) for advanced prostatic cancer.

Anatomy of the pelvic lymphatics

The common iliac nodes are grouped around the artery inferior to the aortic bifurcation and anterior to the fifth lumbar vertebra of sacral promontory. They drain the external and internal iliac nodes and send efferents to the lateral aortic nodes. The common iliac nodes are usually in medial, lateral and intermediate (anterior) chains, the lateral being the main route (Fig. 12.1).

The external iliac nodes are arranged in three subgroups: lateral, medial and anterior to the external iliac vessels; the anterior is inconstant. The medial nodes are considered the main channel of drainage,

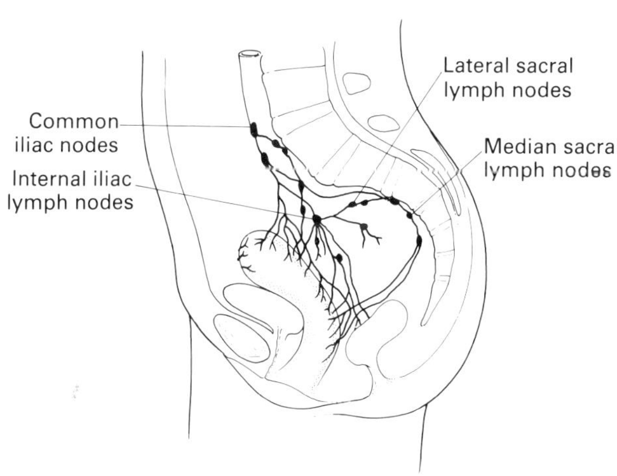

Fig. 12.1 Lymphatic drainage from the female pelvis.

collecting from the inguinal nodes, the deeper layers of the infra-umbilical abdominal wall, the adductor region of the thigh, the glans penis or clitoris, the membranous urethra, the prostate, the vesical fundus, the cervix, uteri and upper vagina. Their efferents pass to the common iliac nodes.

Inferior epigastric and circumflex iliac nodes are associated with their vessels and drain the corresponding areas, being outlying members of the external iliac group and inconstant in number. The internal iliac nodes surround the vessels, receiving afferents from all the pelvic viscera, deep parts of the perineum and gluteal and posterior femoral muscles. Efferents pass to the common iliac nodes. Sacral nodes along the median and lateral sacral vessels, and an obturator node sometimes occurring in the obturator canal, are outlying members of the internal iliac group.

There is considerable bypassing in the iliac groups of lymph nodes. Lymphangiographic studies have demonstrated the connections between the right and left groups.

Bladder

Bladder lymphatics begin in the mucus, intramuscular and extramuscular plexuses. Collecting vessels, which nearly all end in the external iliac nodes, are in three sets: vessels from the trigone emerge on the vesical exterior to run superolaterally; those from the superior surface converge to the posterolateral angle and pass superolaterally across the lateral umbilical ligament to the external iliac nodes (one may go to the internal or common iliac group); those from the inferolateral surface tend to join those from the superior surface. Minute nodules of lymphoid tissue may occur along the vesical lymph vessels.

The ductus deferens, seminal vesicle and prostate

Collecting vessels from the ductus end in the external iliac nodes while those from the seminal vesicle go to the internal and external iliac nodes. Prostatic vessels end mainly in internal iliac and sacral nodes; a vessel from the posterior surface accompanies the vesical vessels to the external iliac nodes and one from the anterior surface gains the internal iliac group by joining vessels of the membranous urethra.

Uterus and cervix

Uterine lymphatics are superficial and deep in the uterine wall. Collecting vessels from the cervix pass laterally in the perimetrium to the external iliac nodes, posterolaterally to the internal iliac nodes and posteriorly to the sacrogenital fold to the rectal and sacral nodes. Some cervical efferents may reach the obturator gluteal nodes. Vessels from the lower part of the uterine body pass mostly to the external iliac nodes with those from the cervix. From the upper part of the body, the fundus and the ureterine tubes, vessels accompany those with the ovaries to the lateral aortic and preaortic nodes, a few passing to the external iliac nodes. The region surrounding the isthmic part of the ureterine tube is drained along the round ligament the superficial inguinal nodes.

Although various sentinel nodes have been described for particular pelvic cancers, it can be seen from the above that reasonable samples of nodal tissue must be taken from the obturator/internal-iliac and external-iliac node groups, and on both sides, to provide a sensitive regional node staging of prostatic, bladder, uterine and cervical cancer.

The extent of the dissection

The extent of the dissection recommended in a laparoscopic pelvic lymphadenectomy is based on the expected lymphatic drainage of a pelvic cancer. It is also influenced by the historical development of the open pelvic lymphadenectomy. The earlier approach of such an open lymphadenectomy was an extensive dissection lateral to the genitofemoral nerve, taking all fibro-lymphatic tissue off the external iliac vessels, extending proximally to the common iliac vessels and medially to skeletonize the obturator vessels and nerve, as well as the internal iliac artery and branches. Finally, the dissection included the presacral and lateral sacral lymph nodes. The distal extent of the dissection included Cloquet's inguinal node and extended inferiorly to the point where the circumflex vein crosses over the external iliac artery (Golimbu *et al.* 1979).

Over the last 10 years, many urological surgeons, at least, have become less radical and have recommended a modified open pelvic lymphadenectomy that includes primarily the nodal and fibro-fatty tissue within the obturator fossa surrounding the obturator vessels and nerve. The lateral and medial borders of this dissection include the external iliac vein and hypogastric artery respectively. The cranial and cordal limits are the bifurcation of the iliac vessels and Cloquet's node or Cooper's ligament respectively.

A major reason in urology for this modification was that 86–94% of the positive nodes from prostate cancer were within the region of the obturator and internal-iliac artery, with no more than 6–14% of cases showing skip lesions, involving only the presacral or common iliac regions (Flocks *et al.* 1959). A second reason is that postoperative complications are more significant, especially when followed by radiotherapy (Paulson *et al.* 1982). Developments such as these in open surgery have influenced our technique for the laparoscopic pelvic lymphadenectomy.

Instrumentation

1 High-flow carbon dioxide insufflator
2 CCD camera and at least one monitor
3 0° 10mm laparoscope (30° optional)
4 Four 10mm ports (trocars/cannulae) with converters for smaller instruments
5 Laparoscopic scissors (with diathermy connection)
6 Two laparoscopic tissue-holding forceps
7 Laparoscopic dissecting forceps
8 Vein or fan retractor
9 Two retrieval bags
10 Endoclip* Applier

Technique

1 Under a general anaesthetic with muscle paralysis and assisted ventilation, the patient is put in a supine position with a 20–25° head-down tilt. A catheter is not required if the patient's bladder has recently emptied and the length of the procedure is expected to be less than 90 minutes. Hip flexion is not required. Heparinization is not recommended but thrombo-embolic deterrent stockings should be worn for DVT (deep venous thrombosis) prophylaxis.

2 Formation of the pneumoperitoneum: the Veress needle is inserted at a 45° angle into the empty pelvis. The position should be checked by aspiration and infusion of 5ml of saline, and the intra-abdominal pressure must be carefully observed to be below 12mm of mercury during insufflation. In the hands of inexperienced laparoscopists, disposable Veress needles with a safety shield are safer. Previous major abdominal surgery is a relative contraindication to blind needle insertion and a Hasson cut-down technique should be used for the first port. This should be inserted well away from a scar so that adhesions can be seen and taken down.

3 Four 10mm ports are placed according to the diagram (Fig. 12.2). The subumbilical port is used for the telescope. The two lateral ports along the edge of the rectus sheath are for manipulative and dissecting instruments. The central port 3–4 cm above the symphysis pubis is for the Endoclip Applier. The ports should be fixed with either grips or purse-string sutures. The universal use of 10mm ports allows greater options for introducing the telescope, Endoclip Applier and 10mm instruments.

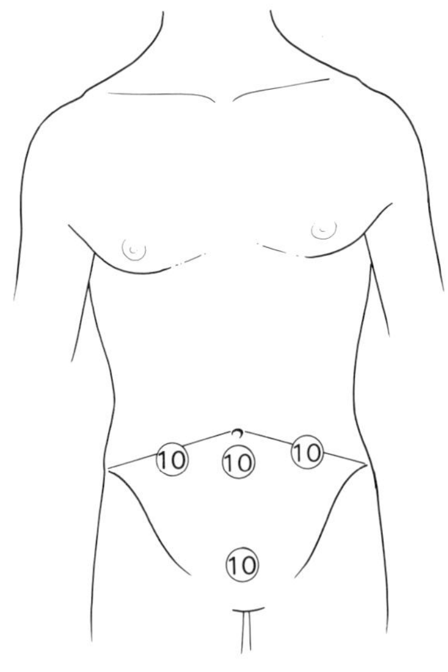

Fig. 12.2 The four 10mm port sites for a laparoscopic pelvic lymphadenectomy.

*A trademark of the United States Surgical Corporation (AutoSuture).

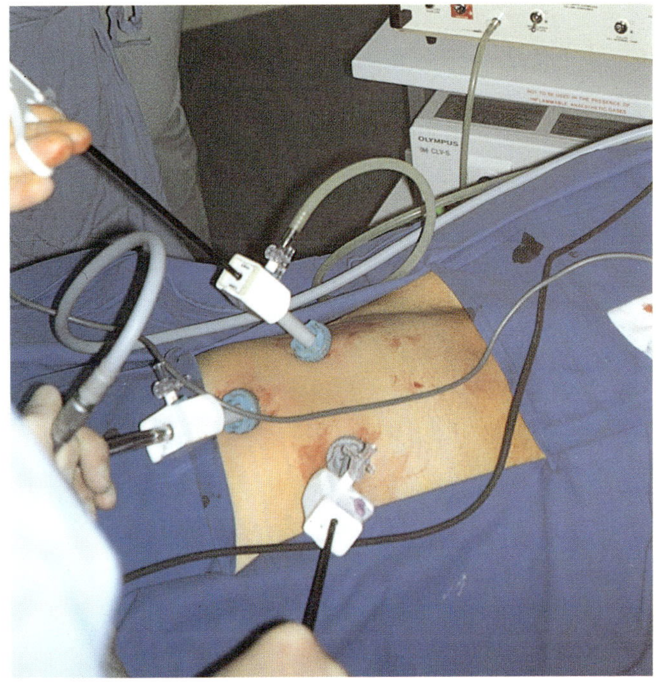

Fig. 12.3 Overview of ports used for a laparoscopic pelvic lymphadenectomy.

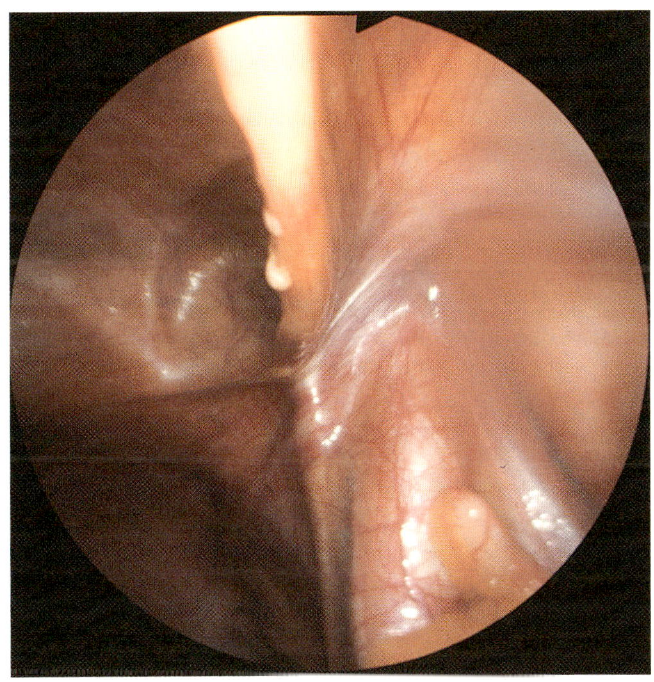

Fig 12.4 An endoscopic view of the left side of the pelvis prior to a laparoscopic pelvic lymphdenectomy.

4 The operator stands on the contralateral side of the patient, the camera-holder on the ipsilateral side (Figs. 11.2, 12.3).

5 Monitors should be at the bottom corners of the operating table.

6 The landmarks of dissection are the umbilical ligament medially, the pubic bone anteriorly and the external iliac vessels laterally (Fig. 12.4). The vas or round ligament courses across this triangle and sometimes requires division for easier access to the obturator fossa.

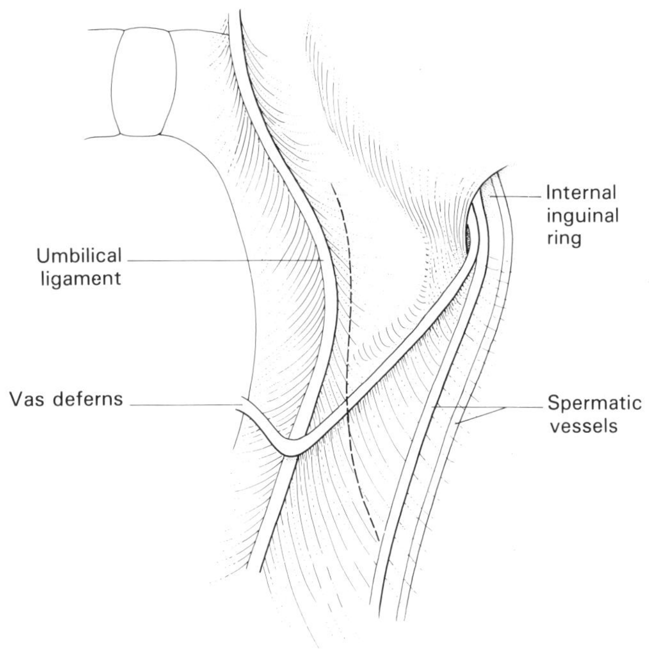

Fig 12.5 Anatomy of a laparoscopic pelvic lymphadenectomy showing the peritoneal incision.

7 The dissection is begun by incising the peritoneum along the medial border of the external iliac vein (Fig. 12.5), and fibro-fatty tissue is removed from around this vessel until it can be clearly exposed between the inguinal ligament and a region 2–3 cm proximal to its bifurcation. The dissection then begins in the obturator fossa and all fibro-fatty tissue is removed until the obturator nerve is exposed (Fig. 12.6). The obturator artery and vein can usually be left intact. The circumflex vein and an aberrant obturator artery (10%) sometimes run across this space and these usually have to be clipped and cut. Minimize the use of diathermy in the obturator fossa to prevent obturator nerve injury.

The dissection always stays lateral to the medial umbilical ligament, and care must be taken closer to the iliac bifurcation, where the ureter is crossed by the ligament. Many of the lymphatics are small and can be sealed with diathermy but larger vessels require clips. Ideally, the fibro-fatty tissue will have been removed in discrete blocks but sometimes this comes away in several pieces. The number of pieces should be noted by a nurse and they can be left to one side in the paracolic gutter until they are all placed in a retrieval bag.

8 The fibro-fatty tissue dissected should be placed in a retrieval bag inserted through a port from the opposite iliac fossa. The neck can be held open with two sets of forceps whilst a third places the tissue inside the bag. Specialized bags are available but the finger of a surgeon's glove suffices. It is advisable to mark the retrieval bags as left and right for future audit of the dissection.

9 Irrigate and aspirate both sites. If there is any oozing, a swab can

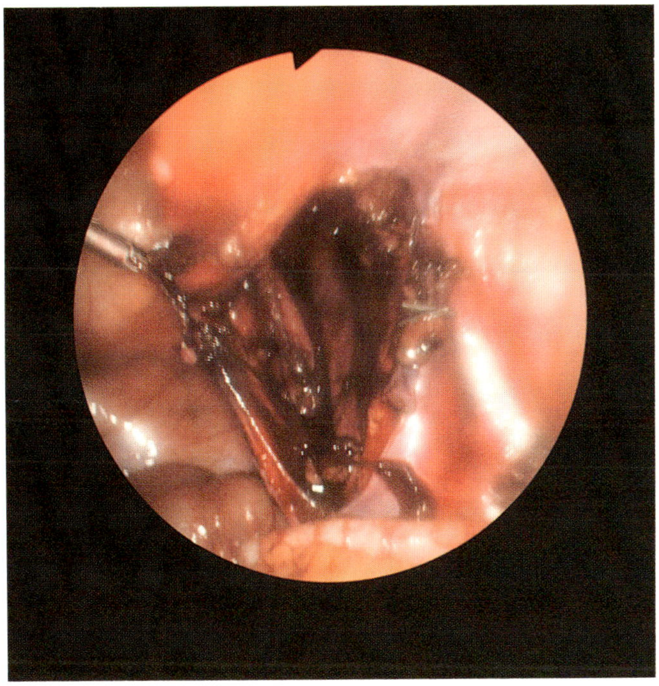

Fig. 12.6 An endoscopic view of the external iliac vein and obturator fossa, from which the lymphatic tissue has been sampled.

be pressed over the affected area. A drain is normally not necessary.

10 After completing the dissection on the opposite side, by the same method, the instruments can be removed and the ports taken out under direct vision. All carbon dioxide is evacuated.

11 To prevent wound-herniation, all wounds require a deep fascial suture. The skin can be sutured with a subcuticular absorbable suture or steristripped. The patients require two or three hours to recover and can usually then be discharged if they can demonstrate effective micturition and do not feel discomfort or nausea.

Complications

The laparoscopic pelvic lymphadenectomy can usually be carried out as a day-case procedure. Only 6% of the patients in King's College Hospital have required overnight stay. The reason was persistent nausea. Some of our early patients received peroperative opiate analgesia and this was identified as a cause of their nausea. Further eradication of this problem has come with the introduction of Ondansetron. This is not given routinely but only to those patients who still feel nauseous two or three hours after their procedure. Complications can otherwise be general to laparoscopy and specific to this procedure.

General complications

Of the reported series of the laparoscopic pelvic lymphadenectomy, only Winfield *et al.* (1992), Ruckle *et al.* (1992) and King's College

Hospital have reported complications. There have been no Veress needle or trocar injuries, probably because of the universal use of disposable equipment with safety shields. Carbon dioxide absorption is less of a problem because the procedures are not overlong. Many elderly patients who have had previous abdominal surgery have adhesions in both iliac fossae and, in particular, on the left side to the sigmoid colon. The inexperienced surgeon may find these prevent safe dissection but, with experience, division of such adhesions merely adds some 20–30 minutes to the procedure. Patients who require division of multiple adhesions usually cannot be discharged as day cases.

Specific complications

Ruckle reported a 14% specific complication rate which included two patients with a DVT, an obturator nerve palsy, a retroperitoneal abscess and an accidental cystotomy. The King's College Hospital experience of this procedure has an 8% complication rate. DVTs have not been experienced in our series possibly due to the universal use of thrombo-embolic deterrent stockings.

One patient required immediate open exploration because of arterial bleeding during dissection. This was identified at the junction between the supposedly obliterated umbilical artery and the internal iliac artery. It was a reminder not to take the dissection so proximally in future, as this is also the point at which the ureter may be cut accidentally, where it crosses beneath the obliterated umbilical artery. Winfield *et al.* (1992) reported a 6% incidence of peroperative haemorrhage. Two of these four cases required urgent exploration. This slightly high incidence probably reflects the variety in radicalism of the lymphadenectomy. The morbidity of a laparoscopic pelvic lymphadenectomy is, however, much less than an open procedure (McCullough *et al.* 1977, Winfield *et al.* 1992).

One King's College Hospital patient went into urinary retention, and this will always be a possibility if routine catheterization is used in elderly men. One would have imagined that carbon dioxide absorption through the dissection sites would be high but the continual measurement of end-tidal carbon dioxide levels and correction with assisted ventilation has not led to any such complications. Minor complications such as the formation of a pneumoscrotum do occur occasionally but these all settle within a few hours of the procedure and do not seem to cause the patient any discomfort.

Discussion

Extraperitoneal staging of pelvic nodes

There is an alternative option for minimally invasive staging of the pelvic nodes, and that is by way of an extraperitoneal pelviscopy (Shafik 1990, 1992, Hald & Rasmussen 1990). The Veress needle in this procedure is placed suprapubically but extraperitoneally. The extraperitoneal space can be easily insufflated, but its lateral restriction is at the point of the deep inguinal ring, and dissection in this area is possibly more difficult than during a transperitoneal approach. Shafik describes a novel approach whereby the telescope is actually introduced through a second incision over the superficial inguinal ring and passed through the inguinal canal to enter the pelvis through the deep inguinal ring. The number of lymph nodes removed with this alternative technique and the sensitivity and specificity are comparable to all reports of the transperitoneal laparoscopic pelvic lymphadenectomy.

One theoretical advantage of this extraperitoneal technique is the ability to come back for a second look if neoadjuvant treatment is commenced. This second look would probably be impossible through the same portal of entry but one could then revert easily to a transperitoneal approach. Unfortunately, once a transperitoneal laparoscopic pelvic lymphadenectomy has been undertaken, there are significant adhesions to the sites of dissection which preclude a second-look dissection by either a transperitoneal or extraperitoneal route.

One of the greatest complications of an extraperitoneal approach is lymphocele formation. This occurs in approximately 10% of patients and requires some form of percutaneous drainage postoperatively. This complication does not occur with the transperitoneal approach because the lymph drains into the open peritoneal cavity and is immediately absorbed.

The representation but not the completeness of this extraperitoneal approach has been shown. Both Winfield (Winfield *et al.* 1992) and Coptcoat (Coptcoat & Wickham 1992) assessed the validity of their transperitoneal laparoscopic procedure in 26 out of 66 and 31 out of 34 cases respectively. Some extranodal tissue was then removed at open dissection, especially at the iliac bifurcation but the false-negative rate was 4% and 0% respectively.

Gynaecological applications

Previous reports of open staging lymphadenectomy in gynaecological cancer have shown a substantial disparity between the clinical and surgical disease extent. This has been reported as a 42% difference for carcinoma of the cervix (La Polla *et al.* 1986) and 52% with carcinoma of the endometrium (Cowles *et al.* 1985). Querleu *et al.* (1991) has reported a series of 39 patients in whom a laparoscopic pelvic lymphadenectomy was performed in the staging of early carcinoma of the cervix. The accuracy of a negative laparoscopic lymphadenectomy and the sensitivity was 100% in this series. The risk of 'skip' metastases (primitive iliac or para-aortic nodes without pelvic node involvement) is less than 2% (Dargent & Salvat 1989) and seems to occur only in patients with large tumour volumes.

The introduction of minimally invasive staging of pelvic lymphadenectomy in itself allows less open curative surgery to be used for early cervical cancer (stage 1, 2a or 2b) with negative nodes. These can probably be cured by vaginal surgery alone or by brachytherapy without the need for external radiotherapy. On the other hand, radical hysterectomy does not now seem justified when positive nodes are known to be present (Potter *et al.* 1990). The consequent reduction of risk and cost justifies the additional general anaesthesia and the short hospital stay of a diagnostic laparoscopy.

Patients with positive nodes should not now have inappropriate and unnecessary extensive surgery or radiotherapy but, as with bladder cancer, this unfortunate group of patients do not yet have any reasonable treatment available. We await the refinement of neoadjuvant and adjuvant chemotherapy regimes which will give this group of node-positive patients a chance of cure.

Some stage 1aII cervical carcinomas without pelvic node metastases can be treated by cervical conization alone. When hysterectomy is not necessary for local control of such tumours, laparoscopic lymphadenectomy helps identify women of reproductive age with micro-invasive carcinomas who may benefit from conservative therapy. The rare cases with no metastases, which justify a radical treatment protocol, can be differentiated from cases with negative nodes, in which cervical conization with preservation of fertility is an acceptable treatment.

Lymph-node metastases in prostatic cancer

The laparoscopic pelvic lymphadenectomy has had its greatest impact in cases of prostatic cancer. The incidence of lymph node metastases in patients who are thought otherwise to have confined localized prostate cancer and are eligible for radical prostatectomy is in the region of 20–30% (Jewett *et al.* 1972, McCullough *et al.* 1974). The likelihood of positive node metastases correlates with both local tumour volume and the degree of differentiation (Barzell *et al.* 1977).

Prostatic specific antigen (PSA) levels between 20 and 50 ng/ml usually have a 65% risk of nodal metastases or seminal vesicle involvement (Hudson *et al.* 1992). This latter finding has led us to develop the following protocol for patients with localized prostate cancer. A patient with a PSA level over 20 ng/ml who would still have been considered for radical surgery will undergo a staging pelvic lymphadenectomy as a separate day-case procedure. The likelihood of positive nodes is high and patients are unlikely to experience the psychological trauma of recovering to find that their definitive procedure has not gone ahead. Patients with a PSA level lower than this will undergo a laparoscopic pelvic lymphadenectomy under the same anaesthetic as their planned definitive surgery. Frozen sections will be sent and the most likely outcome is that the sections will be negative and definitive surgery can go ahead.

The only concern with this protocol is that frozen sections have a false-negative rate of up to 19% and are not as reliable as paraffin sections for the diagnosis of micrometastases (Catalona & Stein 1982). The obvious advantages of only one anaesthetic outweigh this when positive nodes are unlikely to be found. It must be stressed that such a protocol is only used after CT or MRI scanning of the abdomen and pelvis. There is absolutely no point in carrying out a laparoscopic pelvic lymphadenectomy when macroscopically enlarged nodes can be identified on noninvasive scans.

Such nodes can be easily assessed with fine needle aspiration (Correa *et al.* 1981). The role of the laparoscopic lymphadenectomy is in those cases where either CT or MRI is negative for nodes.

The laparoscopic pelvic lymphadenectomy has also changed the type of curative surgery that can be offered to the patient. The radical perineal prostatectomy was first described by Young (1905) but has not gained wide acceptance because a staging open pelvic lymphadenectomy required an extra-abdominal incision. Thus the standard form of radical prostate surgery has become the radical retropubic prostatectomy as pioneered by Walsh (Walsh *et al.* 1983). Now that we can stage pelvic lymphadenectomy laparoscopically, there is no need to continue with the retropubic dissection. The perineal approach is much less invasive, is associated with much less blood loss, is still nerve-preserving and in many series no blood transfusion is used at all (Frazier *et al.* 1992). Patients can be discharged three or four days earlier with this type of surgery and this will probably become the standard method now that a laparoscopic pelvic lymphadenectomy is gaining acceptance for its accuracy and specificity of node sampling.

It is therefore interesting to see the impact of minimally invasive surgical procedures not just as a technique in itself but as part of the overall surgical management of a patient. Patients with positive nodes receive hormonal manipulation which some hope may be neoadjuvant with regard to a possible curative radical prostatectomy. We know that early endocrine management instituted at the time of surgery can delay progression of known positive nodes from 20 months to an average of 60 months (Zincke *et al.* 1986). What is required in these cases is a technique for second-look node staging after neoadjuvant treatment and this takes us back to our point above concerning the possible role of an extraperitoneal route. The laparoscopic pelvic lymphadenectomy is feasible and does not seem to carry any additional morbidity after radiotherapy (Winfield *et al.* 1992) which also points to a role for second-look management.

Laparoscopic lymphadenectomy and bladder cancer

The role of the laparoscopic pelvic lymphadenectomy for bladder cancer is still unclear. Few people have evaluated this because of the absence of any satisfactory treatment when positive nodes are found (Dretler *et al.* 1973).

However, this argument is parallel to that in gynaecological cancers, and surely the opportunity to prevent patients going through inappropriate and unnecessary surgery or radiotherapy must make this staging procedure worthwhile.

Skinner (1982) and Malkowicz (Malkowicz *et al.* 1991) have argued that micrometastases in the pelvic nodes do not make any difference to overall survival following a radical cystectomy, but Malkowicz's series only contains 11 patients, and it is difficult to understand why nodal metastatic bladder cancer would behave in such a tolerant way compared with other pelvic cancers. Again, our hope would be that positive nodes would indicate the use of neoadjuvant chemotherapy followed by a second-look sampling and radical surgery if the nodes become negative. This is still very speculative, but we should have some answers within the next few years.

Finding positive nodes during a radical prostatectomy is actually much less common than finding either prostatic capsular involvement or seminal vesicle involvement. Understaging in these two respects has caused great concern, and it is now possible to carry the laparoscopic dissection down through the pouch of Douglas towards the seminal vesicles and lateral and posterior aspects of the prostatic capsule. Biopsies can be taken from these regions which should allow us to stage the local prostate cancer more correctly.

The operation is therefore developing into a synchronous combined laparoscopic and radical perineal prostatectomy in the same way that the synchronous combined abdominoperineal resection for low rectal cancers developed. We have carried out four such procedures and although the operative time for the staging laparoscopy was extended by up to an average of 60 minutes, the information from negative vesicle and capsular biopsies made the subsequent radical prostatectomy much more certain of cure.

This is probably the way that all staging lymphadenectomies for pelvic cancer will go, in that either the whole or parts of the definitive curative surgery will be undertaken in the same minimally invasive way.

The laparoscopic pelvic lymphadenectomy can be successfully undertaken as a day-case procedure provided that there are no other medical or social problems. We have preferred to carry this out as a

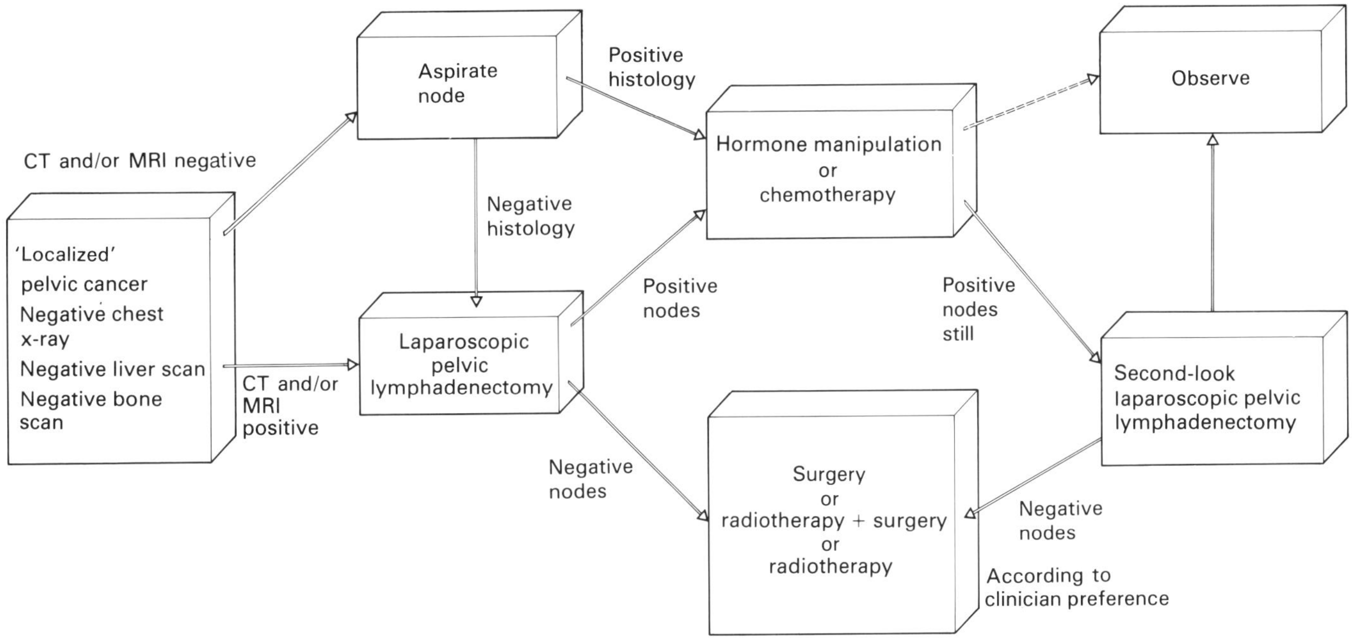

Fig. 12.7 An algorithm for the possible future staging of pelvic cancers in association with neoadjuvant treatment.

separate day-case procedure because the planning of definitive surgery becomes much more precise when the patients has already been staged. This concept has also been supported by the patients, who appreciate knowing whether curative surgery will be undertaken when their procedure commences.

In conclusion, one can say already that the laparoscopic pelvic lymphadenectomy is accurate and sensitive for the staging of lymph nodes affected by micrometastases from all pelvic cancers. Its value at the present time lies in staging rather than in therapy but as the laparoscopic techniques evolve, it may become part of a curative surgical procedure, as in the case of the superior dissection of the prostate prior to a radical perineal prostatectomy and reanastomosis. Any staging lymphadenectomy will only be worthwhile if the finding of micrometastases does alter the management of any particular patient. This is certainly true in early cervical cancer and prostate cancer but we still await a refinement of neoadjuvant chemotherapy and/or radiotherapy for bladder cancer and for more advanced endometrial cancer before the true impact in these cases will be felt. In these cases, a second-look node sampling will be required and a combination of preliminary laparoscopic extraperitoneal and secondary transperitoneal procedures may be considered (Fig. 12.7). The laparoscopic pelvic lymphadenectomy is a simple, safe day-case procedure that surgically stages pelvic cancer.

References

Bagshaw M.A., Ray G.R., Cox R.S. (1987) Selecting initial therapy for prostate cancer: Radiation therapy perspective. *Cancer*, **60**, 521.

Barzell W., Bean M.A., Hilaris B.S., Whitmore W.F. Jr. (1977) Prostatic adenocarcinoma: Relationship of grade and local extent to the pattern of metastases. *Journal of Urology*, **118**, 278.

Benson K.H., Watson R.A., Spring D.B., Agee R.E. (1981) The value of computerised tomography in evaluation of pelvic lymph nodes. *Journal of Urology*, **126**, 63.

Catalona W.J. & Stein A.J. (1982) Accuracy of frozen section detection of lymph node metastases in prostatic carcinoma. *Journal of Urology*, **127**, 460.

Coptcoat M.J. & Wickham J.E.A. (1992) Laparoscopy in Urology. *Minimally Invasive Therapy*, **1**, 337–42.

Correa R.S. Jr., Kidd C.R., Burnett L., Brannen G.E, Gibbons R.P., Cummings K.B. (1981) Percutaneous pelvic lymph node aspiration in carcinoma of the prostate. *Journal of Urology*, **126**, 190.

Cowles T.A., Magrina J.F., Masterson B.J., Capen C.V. (1985) Comparison of clinical and surgical staging in patients with endometrial carcinoma. *Obstetrics and Gynaecology*, **66**, 413.

Dargent D. & Salvat J. (1989) *L'envahissement ganglionnaire pelvien*. MEDSI, Paris.

Dretler S.P., Ragsdale B.D., Leadbetter W.F. (1973) The value of pelvic lymphadenectomy in the surgical treatment of bladder cancer. *Journal of Urology*, **109**, 414.

Feigen M., Crocker E.F., Read J., Crandon A. J. (1987) The value of lymphoscitingraphy, lymphangiography and computer tomography scanning in the preoperative assessment of lymph nodes involved by pelvic malignant conditions. *Surgery, Gynaecology and Obstetrics*, **165**, 107–10.

Flocks R.H., Culp D., Porto R. (1959) Lymphatic spread from prostate cancer. *Journal of Urology*, **81**, 194.

Frazier H.A., Robertson J.E., Paulson D.E. (1992) Radical prostatectomy: The pros and cons of the perineal versus retropubic approach. *Journal of Urology*, **147**, 888–90.

Gershman A., Daykhovsky L., Chandra M., Danoff D., Grundfest W. (1990) Laparoscopic pelvic lymphadenectomy. Journal of Laparoendoscopic *Surgery*, **1**:1, 63–8.

Golimbu M., Morales P., Al-Askari S., Brown J. (1979) Extended pelvic lymphadenectomy for prostatic cancer. *Journal of Urology*, **121**, 617.

Hald T. & Rasmussen F. (1990) Extraperitoneal pelviscopy: A new aid in staging of lower urinary tract tumours; a preliminary report. *Journal of Urology*, **124**, 245.

Hudson M.A., Bahnson R.B., Catalona W.J. (1992) Clinical use of prostate and specific antigen in patients with prostate cancer. *Journal of Urology*, **142**, 1011.

Jewett H.J., Eggleston J.C., Yawn D.H. (1972) Radical prostatectomy in the management of carcinoma of the prostate: Probable causes of some therapeutic failures. *Journal of Urology*, **107**, 1034.

La Polla J.P., Schlaerth J.B., Gaddis O., Morrow C.P. (1986) The influence of surgical staging on the evaluation and treatment of patients with cervical carcinoma. *Gynaecology and Oncology*, **24**, 194.

Loening S.A., Schmidt J.D., Brown R.C., Hawtry C.E., Fallon B., Culp D.A. (1977) A comparison between lymphangiography and pelvic lymph node dissection in the staging of prostatic cancer. *Journal of Urology*, **117**, 752.

Malkowicz S.B., Nichols P., Lieskovsky G., Boyd S.D., Huffman J., Skinner D.G. (1991) The role of radical cystectomy in the management of high grade, superficial bladder cancer (PA, P1, PIS and P2). *Journal of Urology*, **144**, 641–5.

McCullough D.L., Prout G.R., Daly J.J. (1974) Carcinoma of the prostate and lymphatic metastases. *Journal of Urology*, **111**, 65.

McCullough D.L., McLaughlin A.P., Gittes R.F. (1977) Morbidity of pelvic lymphadenectomy and radical prostatectomy for prostatic cancer. *Journal of Urology*, **145**, 988–91.

Parra R., Adrus C., Boullier J.A. (1992) Staging laparoscopic pelvic lymph node dissection: Comparison of results with open pelvic lymphadenectomy. *Journal of*

Urology, **147**, 875–8.

Paulson D.F., Lin G.H., Hinshaw W., Stephani S. (1982) The Uro-Oncology Research Group: Radical surgery versus radiotherapy for adenocarcinoma of the prostate. *Journal of Urology*, **128**, 502.

Potter M.E., Alvarez R.D., Shingleton H.M., Soong S.J., Hatch K.D. (1990) Early invasive cervical cancer with pelvic lymph node involvement; to complete or not to complete radical hysterectomy? *Gynaecology and Oncology*, **37**, 78–81.

Querleu D., Leblanc E., Castelain B. (1991) Laparoscopic pelvic lymphadenectomy in the early staging of early carcinoma of the cervix. *American Journal of Obstetrics and Gynaecology*, **164**, 579–81.

Ray G.R., Pistenma D.A., Castellino R.A., Kempson R., Meares E., Bagshaw M.A. (1976) Operative staging of apparently localized adenocarcinoma of the prostate: Results in fifty selected patients 1; experimental design and preliminary results. *Cancer*, **38**, 73.

Rifkin M.C., Zerhouni E.A., Gatsonis C.A. *et al.* (1990) Comparison of magnetic resonance imaging and ultrasonography in staging early prostate cancer. *New England Journal of Medicine*, **323**, 621.

Ruckle H., Hadley R., Lui P., Stewart S. (1992) Laparoscopic pelvic lymph node dissection: Assessment of intraoperative and early post-operative complications. *Journal of Endourology*, **6**: 2, 117–19.

Schuessler W.W., Vancaille T.G., Reich H., Griffith D.P. (1991) Transperitoneal endosurgical lymphadenectomy in patients with localised prostate cancer. *Journal of Urology*, **145**, 988.

Shafik A. (1990) Inguinal pelviscopy: A new approach for examining the pelvic organs. *Gynaecological and Obstetric Investigations*, **30**, 159.

Shafik M.D. (1992) Extraperitoneal laparoscopic lymphadenectomy in prostatic cancer: Preliminary report of a new approach. *Journal of Endourology*, **6**: 2, 113–16.

Skinner D.G. (1982) Management of invasive bladder cancer: A meticulous pelvic node dissection can make a difference. *Journal of Urology*, **128**, 34.

Walsh P.C., Lepos H., Eggleston J.D. (1983) Radical prostatectomy with preservation of sexual function; anatomical and pathological considerations. *Prostate*, **4**, 473.

Winfield H.N., Donovan J.F., See W.A., Loening S.A., Williams R.D. (1992) Laparoscopic pelvic lymph node dissection for genitourinary malignancies: Indications, techniques and results. *Journal of Endourology*, **6**: 2, 103–12.

Young H.H. (1905) The early diagnosis and radical cure of carcinoma of the prostate; being a study of 40 cases and presentation of a radical operation which was carried out in four cases. *Bulletin of the Johns Hopkins Hospital*, **16**, 315.

Zincke H., Fleming T.R., Furlow W.L. *et al.* (1981) Radical retropubic prostatectomy and pelvic lymphadenectomy for high stage cancer of the prostate. *Cancer*, **47**, 1901.

Zincke H., Utz D.C., Taylor W.F. (1986) Bilateral pelvic lymphadenectomy and radical prostatectomy for clinical stage C prostatic cancer; role of adjuvant treatment for residual cancer and in disease progression. *Journal of Urology*, **135**, 1199–205.

13: Laparoscopic Para-Aortic Lymphadenectomy

M. J. COPTCOAT

Introduction

Para-aortic nodal tissue can be removed by either a transperitoneal or retroperitoneal approach. Our experience so far has been to go through the peritoneal cavity using the same position and same basic techniques as for a laparoscopic transperitoneal nephrectomy.

Our interest in this started when a patient was referred with a 3 cm residual nodal mass just beneath the left renal vein following three courses of chemotherapy for testicular cancer (Fig. 13.1). The case was a great success but it was clear that adequate visualization required medial displacement of surrounding structures and that any attempt to remove all postchemotherapy lymphatic tissue would be very difficult, given available instrumentation and restricted angles of access.

Its role therefore lies in association with the philosophy that only significantly enlarged residual tissue should be excised. When such tissue is to be removed, a laparoscopic transperitoneal lymphadenectomy is a very reasonable, safe, minimally invasive alternative to traditional open exploration.

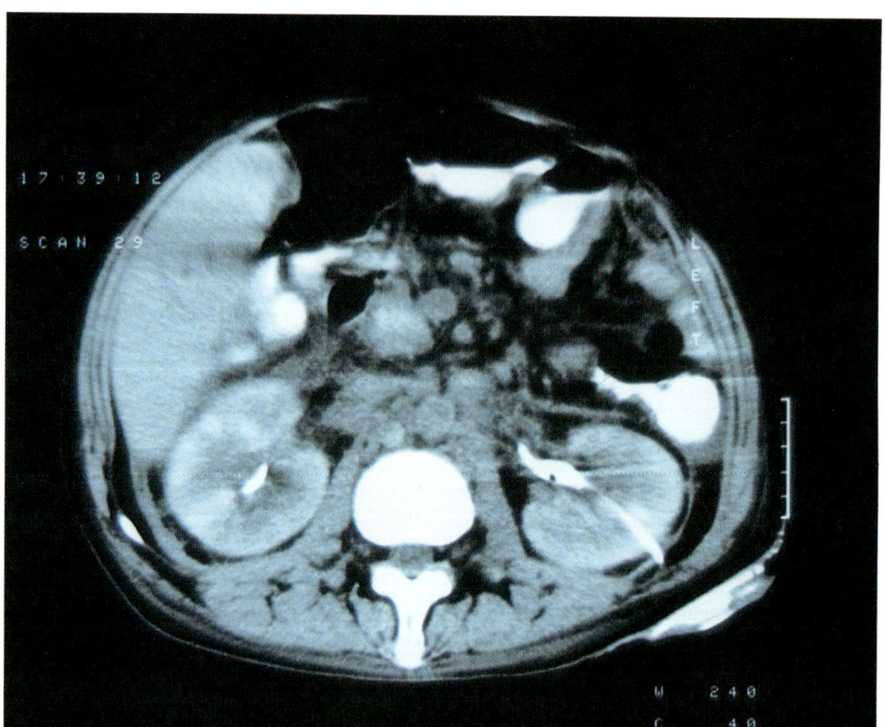

Fig 13.1 A CT scan showing a residual para-aortic lymphatic mass beneath the left renal vein following chemotherapy for a testicular teratoma.

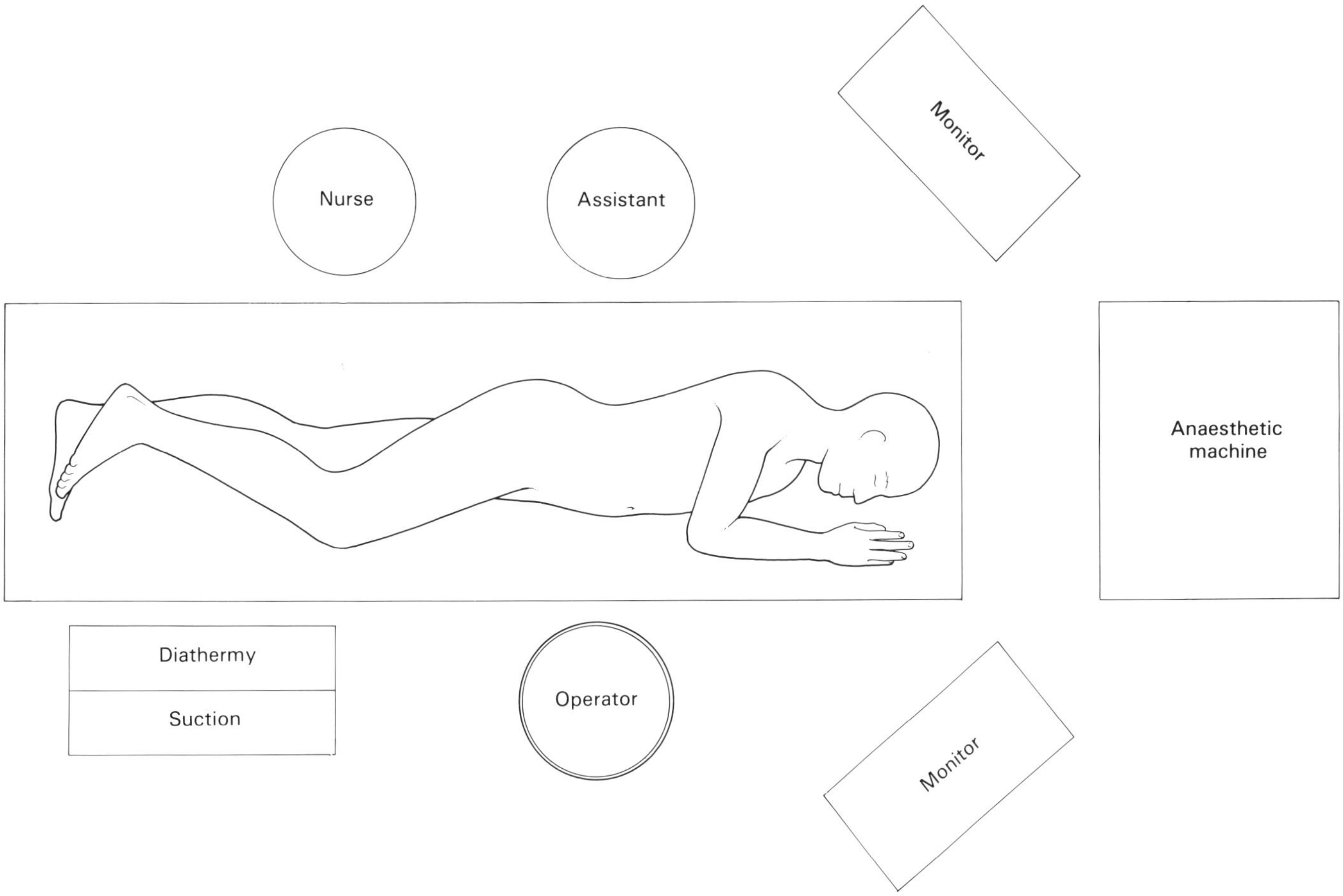

Fig. 13.2 Layout of equipment for a laparoscopic para-aortic lymphadenectomy.

Laparoscopic instrumentation

1 High-flow carbon dioxide insufflator
2 CCD camera and 2 monitors
3 Veress needle (safety type)
4 0° 10mm laparoscope (30° optional)
5 Two 10mm ports with grips and converters/two 5mm downsizers
6 One 12mm port with grips and converters/two 10mm and two 5mm downsizers
7 Laparoscopic scissors (diathermy connection)
8 Laparoscopic dissecting forceps
9 Laparoscopic Babcock grasping forceps
10 Laparoscopic soft grasping forceps
11 Endoclip* Applier (medium/large)
12 Fan retractor
13 Endo GIA* 30 stapler

*A trademark of the United States Surgical Corporation (AutoSuture).

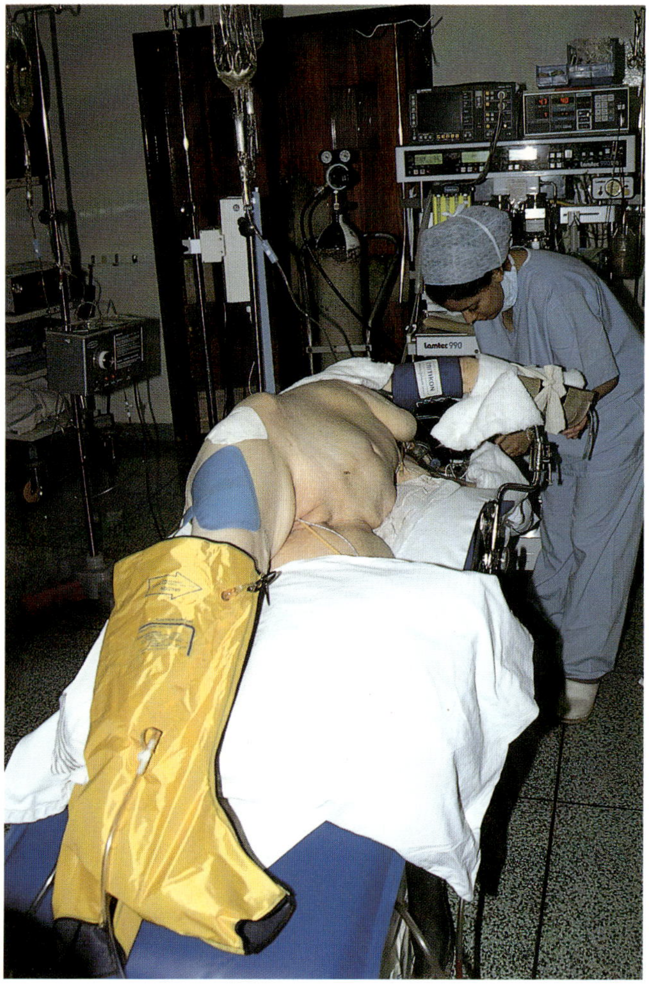

Fig. 13.3 The position of the patient for a laparoscopic para-aortic lymphadenectomy.

Technique

1 Under a general anaesthetic with muscle paralysis and assisted ventilation, the patient is put into a lateral position with the table broken between the ribs and iliac crest (Fig. 13.3). The patient can be held by straps or, preferably, supported on a rest with slight backward tilt. A urethral catheter is required but ureteric intubation is not. Thrombo-embolic deterrent stockings are recommended.

2 The Veress needle is inserted horizontally at the edge of the rectus sheath in line with the umbilicus (Fig. 13.4). This will also be the site for the telescope port. A long needle is required for all but the thinnest patients. The infusion and drop tests are performed to verify correct placement of the Veress needle.

Early insufflation is often prevented by a high intra-abdominal pressure feedback (over 12mmHg), but this is usually due to malpositioning of the needle tip. It is countered by gently lifting the tip up laterally where it becomes free from the colon. Insufflate 2–4 litres of carbon dioxide.

3 The Veress needle is removed. The skin incision is lengthened

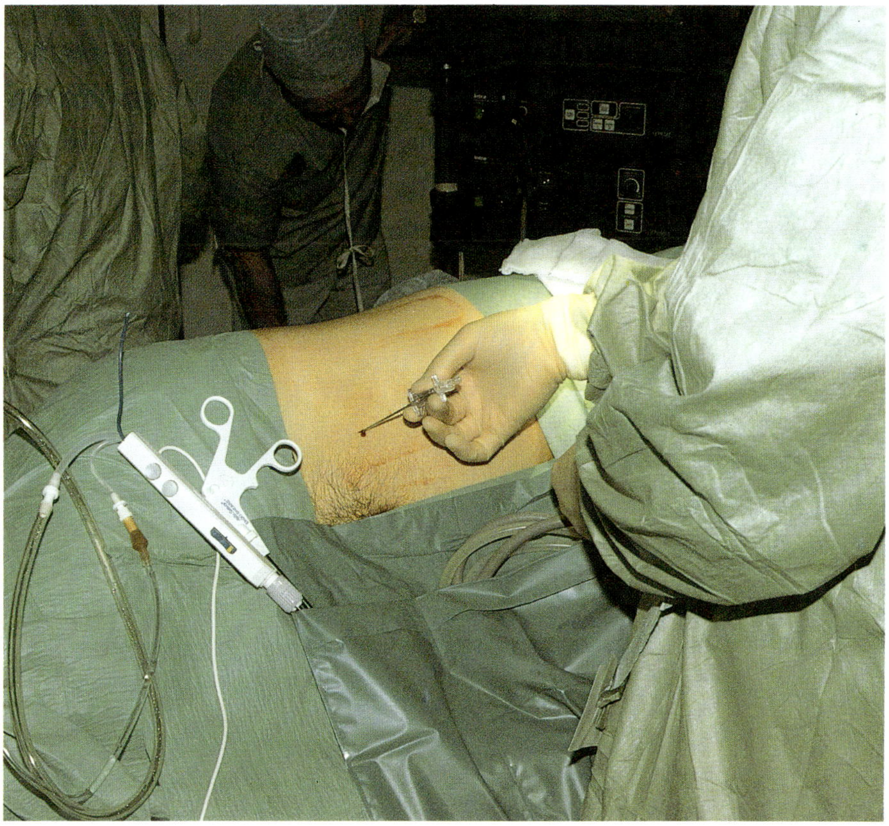

Fig. 13.4 Insertion of the Veress needle at the edge of the rectus sheath.

horizontally to 11 mm and a disposable 10 mm port with grip is inserted (Fig. 13.5). The carbon dioxide is connected to this port until secondary ports have been added.

4 Inspect the abdomen with the laparoscope. Identify the potential sites for secondary ports, which should be well away from superficial vessels. Insert two secondary ports under direct vision in the midclavicular line. These are the principal sites for dissection instruments used by the operator.

Keep the 12 mm port, which is for the potential use of the Endo GIA 30 stapler, at least 2 cm below the ribs to allow greater freedom of movement.

A short interchange of telescope with the larger secondary port will allow visual adjustment of the grip and cannula of the first telescope port. Subsequent carbon dioxide insufflation should be through

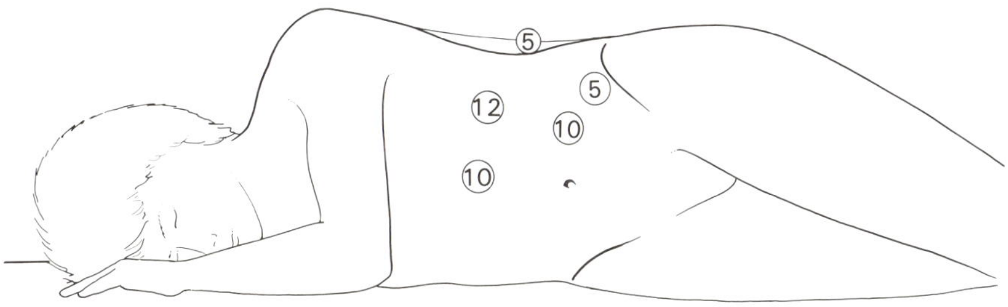

Fig. 13.5 The port sites for a laparoscopic transperitoneal para-aortic lymphadenectomy.

a secondary port to prevent unnecessary local cooling of the telescope. The telescope should be prewarmed to body core temperature.
5 The peritoneal reflection lateral to the colon is incised from the hepatic or splenic flexure down to the pelvic brim (Fig. 15.5). The use of the lateral position facilitates medial displacement of the colon by virtue of gravity. A mild preoperative phosphate enema will also have helped reduce the bulk of the colon.

Although this plane is said to be bloodless, there is often a small artery at either end of the reflection. Together with the usually trivial superficial peritoneal vessels, it will require diathermy haemostasis to prevent small haemorrhages accumulatively absorbing the light. Such oozing is precipitated by vasodilatation caused by local carbon dioxide absorption but is never so severe as to be anything other than a nuisance for camera visualization.
6 A single 5mm port can then be safely placed in the midaxillary line for lateral retraction of tissues. A 10mm port should be placed in the midline half way between the umbilicus and xiphisternum (Fig. 13.5). This port will be used for the fan retractor that will displace the colon medially.

Dissection of the para-aortic tissues is begun at the aortic bifurcation and then proceeds proximally in much the same way as an open lymphadenectomy. It is advisable to have the aspirator within the abdomen all of the time and if all the ports have been used up, an additional 5mm port will be required for this and this can be placed fairly laterally. The vascular supply to nodal tissue can be divided between clips.It is rare for the Endo GIA 30 stapler to be needed but a 12mm port should be at hand.
7 A drain is placed through one of the 5mm port sites to facilitate the rapid removal of carbon dioxide and to provide an indicator for possible haemorrhage. The drain can be removed on the first postoperative day.
8 A fascial suture is required for 10mm and 12mm puncture sites. Steristrips are suitable for some female patients, but generally more active patients are best given a simple 3/0 Ethylon suture to each skin wound.

Discussion

Janetschek has described a series of procedures of a laparoscopic retroperitoneal para-aortic lymphadenectomy on six pigs (Janetschek *et al.* 1992). What impresses me is not so much that this technique was shown to be feasible but that the area of dissection was shown on video to be completely cleared and could be mistaken for that seen after an open lymphadenectomy.

His suggestion that such a laparoscopic technique could be used for para-aortic nodal staging following initial diagnosis of a testicular tumour is quite reasonable but will only find a place with those who do not prefer a more conservative wait and see policy for stage 1 testicular cancer.

References

Janetschek G., Reissigl A., Peschel R., Bartsch G. (1992) Laparoscopic retroperitoneal lymphadenectomy for testicular tumour; Animal studies and first clinical experience. *Minimally Invasive Therapy*, **1**: 1, 68 (B31).

14: Laparoscopic Retroperitoneal Surgery

M.J. COPTCOAT AND C.G. EDEN

Introduction

Retroperitoneal endoscopy is true laparoscopy as defined by its Greek origin in the word *lapros*, which literally translated means 'flank'. Retroperitoneal endoscopy is not new but without the availability of current instrumentation, previous attempts were not often successful. In particular, a retroperitoneal endoscopic ureterolithotomy and pyelolithotomy were abandoned in favour of ureteroscopic and percutaneous intrarenal techniques (Wickham & Miller 1983).

The majority of newly described laparoscopic procedures on retroperitoneal structures have used a transperitoneal approach such as a transperitoneal ureterolysis and transperitoneal nephrectomy. It is only recently that Gaur (1992) has reminded us of a route of access that had always been second nature to us in open surgery. Gaur's contribution has been to introduce the concept of a dissecting balloon that is placed through a small incision into the retroperitoneal space. He in fact used a surgeon's glove that equally sufficed. As the balloon is inflated, the dense areolar tissue binding the retroperitoneal fat is broken down in only a few minutes. A working compartment of up to 2 litres can easily be achieved.

Direct insufflation of carbon dioxide without a balloon had not been successful in our hands because it produced a very uneven compartment still held in places by fibrous septae. The balloon breaks these down but does require high pressures of up to 100ml of mercury. This approach will probably take over for most nephrectomies and ureterolysis for retroperitoneal fibrosis.

The difficult mid- or upper-ureteric stone that is recalcitrant to extracorporeal shockwave lithotripsy, and cannot be reached with a ureteroscope from either above or below, can now be treated by retroperitoneal endoscopy. A pyeloplasty using this approach is also feasible and it may turn out to provide the same excellent results as open pyeloplasty but with the minimal invasiveness and morbidity usually associated with a percutaneous endopyelotomy or pyelolysis, which does not have the same long-term success.

Laparoscopic instrumentation

1 Catheter with Helmstein balloon
2 High-flow carbon dioxide insufflator
3 CCD camera and monitor(s)

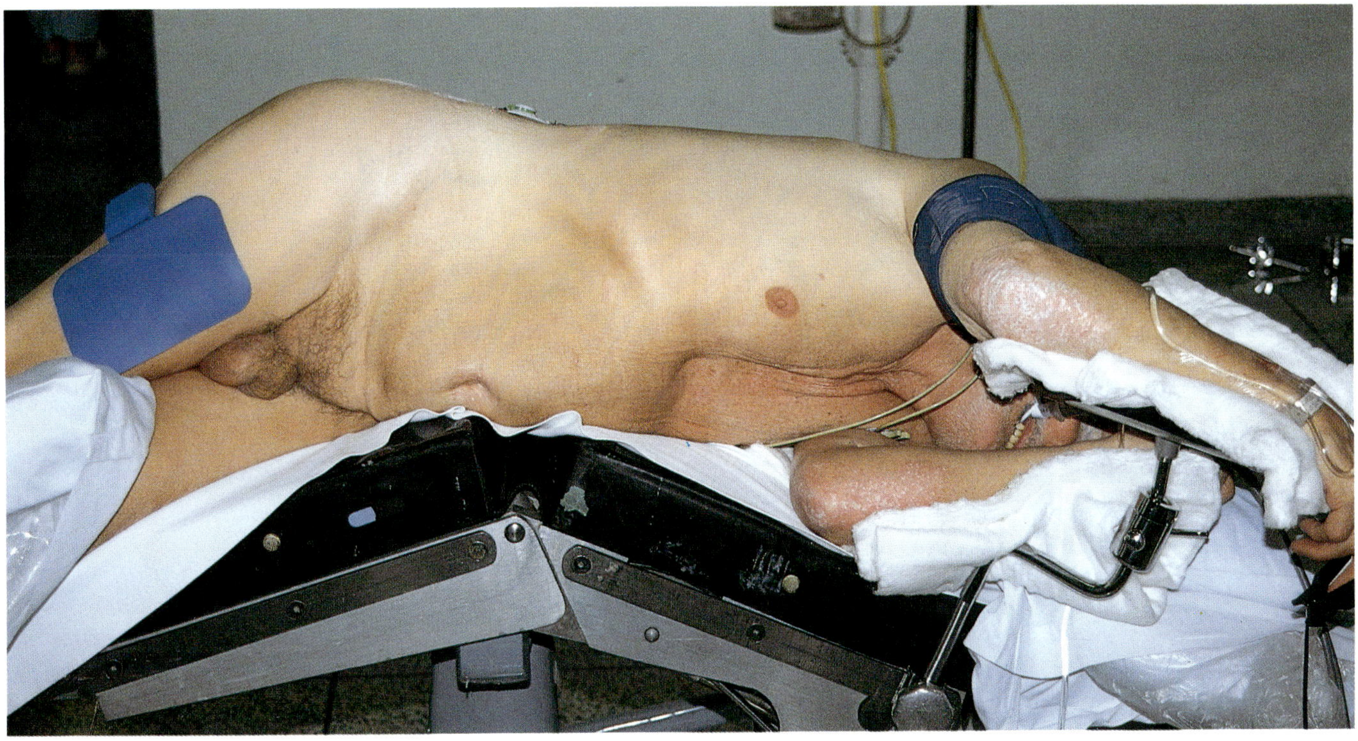

Fig 14.1 Position of the patient for retroperitoneal laparoscopy.

4 One 10mm Hasson port
5 Two 10mm ports (replace with two 12mm ports for a nephrectomy) with converters/downsizers
6 Two 5mm ports
7 Laparoscopic scissors (diathermy connection)
8 Laparoscopic Babcock forceps
9 Laparoscopic dissecting forceps
10 Laparoscopic soft grasping forceps
11 Endoclip* Applier (medium/large)
12 Fan retractor
13 Endo GIA* 30 stapler (for nephrectomy)

Technique

Access to the retroperitoneal space

1 It will be helpful if the relevant ureter is intubated with an indwelling 6 or 7F catheter. This can be taped to an indwelling urethral catheter.
2 Under a general anaesthetic, the patient is placed in the lateral position with the table fully broken (Fig. 14.1). The patient should be supported in the routine way, as for an open retroperitoneal approach.
3 A 2cm transverse incision is made 4cm superior to the anterior

*A trademark of the United States Surgical Corporation (AutoSuture).

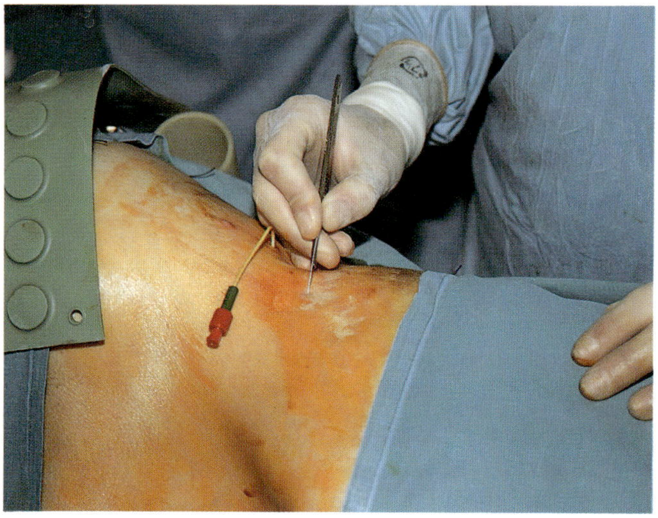

(a)

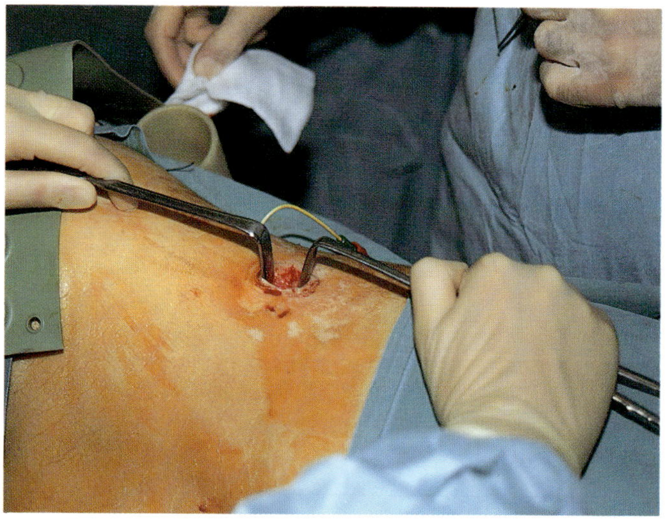

(b)

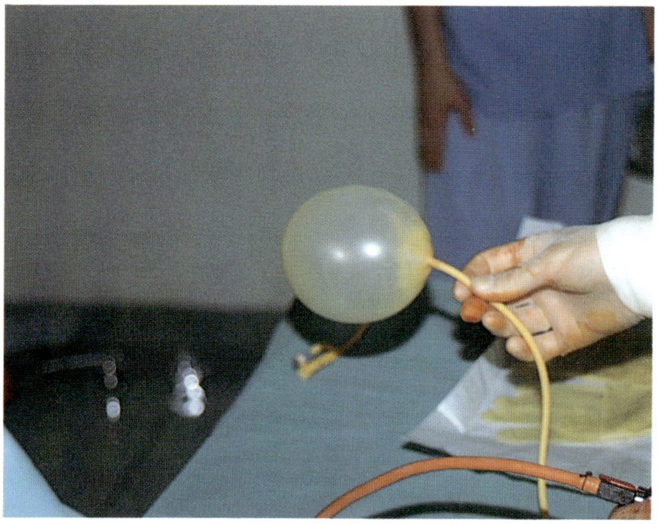

(c)

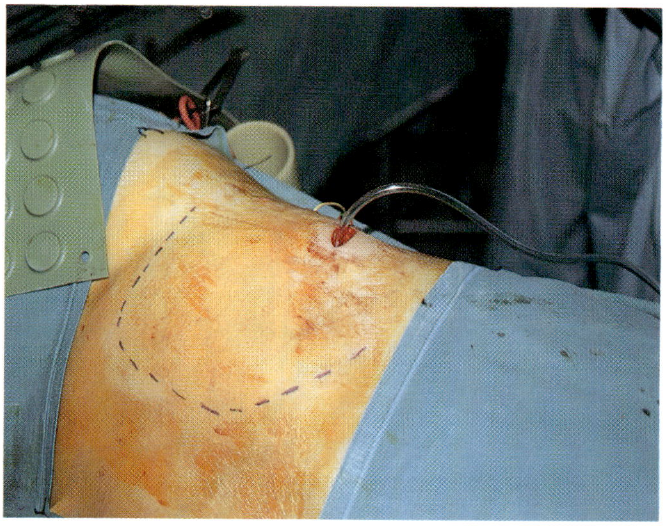

(d)

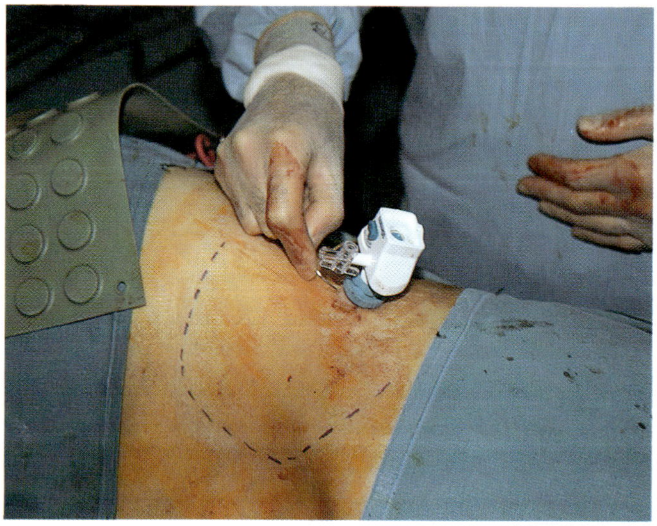

(e)

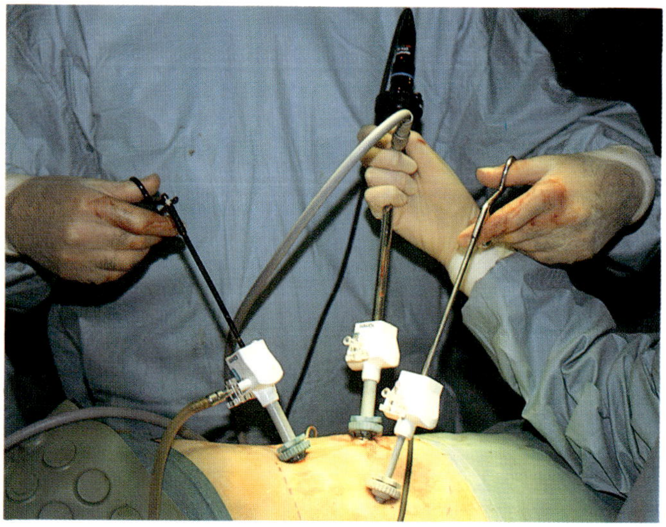

(f)

Fig 14.2 (*opposite*) Retroperitoneal laparoscopy. (a) A 2–2.5 cm transverse incision is made 4 cm above the anterior superior iliac spine. Dissection stops at the peritoneum. (b) Space is created for the Helmstein balloon catheter. (c) The balloon catheter is inflated with air, using a sphygmomanometer insufflator, and tested to a pressure of 100 mmHg. (d) The balloon catheter is reinflated to a volume of 2 litres for 3–5 minutes in the retroperitoneal space and the pressure is monitored closely by means of a side arm to a pressure transducer. The anterior margin of the retroperitoneal space created allows an anteriorly placed port. (e) The blunt Hasson port is inserted through the incision and held with a purse-string suture. (f) An overview of ports used for retroperitoneal laparoscopy.

superior iliac spine (Fig. 14.2a). This is deepened with a gridiron approach (Fig. 14.2b) through the fibres of the anterior abdominal wall until a finger can be gently pushed back over the peritoneum and into the retroperitoneal space.

4 The Helmstein balloon should be checked for integrity up to a pressure of 100 mmHg (Fig. 14.2c). The deflated balloon is then placed into the retroperitoneal space and gradually inflated with a sterilized sphygmomanometer insufflator.

By means of a T tube from the insufflator to a pressure transducer one can monitor the insufflation pressure. The pressure should be kept below 100 mmHg and insufflation should continue until 1.5–2 litres of air has been introduced. There is usually a sharp rise in pressure with inflation, which then rapidly falls as the retroperitoneum is dissected.

The balloon should be inflated at a maximum volume for approximately 3–5 minutes to ensure tamponade of any small vessels which might otherwise bleed (Fig. 14.2d). The balloon is then removed. The working space is created by the balloon at the beginning of the procedure and is simply maintained by subsequent carbon dioxide insufflation. It does not significantly increase, and so care must be taken at this initial stage to ensure that the correct amount of peritoneal reflection has occurred for that particular procedure. This is particularly important for a nephrectomy, where sufficient anterior peritoneal reflection is required to allow access for an anteriorly placed port through which a haemostatic clip or stapler can be introduced perpendicular to the renal pedicle.

Gaur (1992) recommends that the balloon catheter be inflated a second time under the perinephric fascia. This rapidly progresses the dissection, but the plane is not always easy to identify if there has been perinephric inflammation.

5 The blunt Hasson port is inserted through the incision and a purse-string suture holds this in place and creates a fairly air-tight seal (Fig. 14.2e). This will be the port for the telescope.

Carbon dioxide insufflation is set up in the usual way. It is connected initially to this port but will be transferred to secondary ports once these have been inserted. Secondary ports are inserted under direct vision according to the diagram (Fig. 14.3).

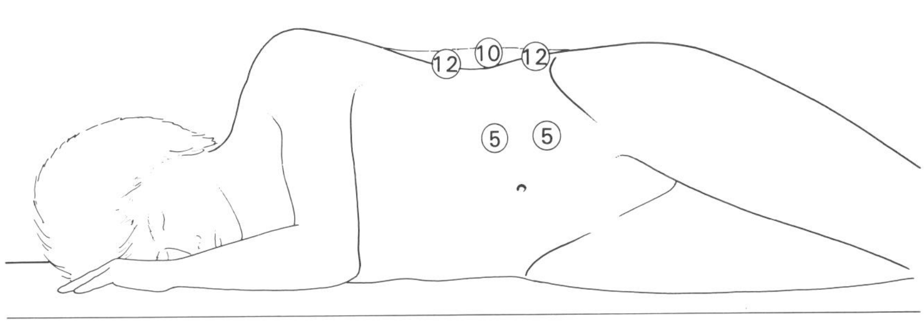

Fig. 14.3 The port sites for a retroperitoneal laparoscopic nephrectomy, pyeloplasty or ureterolithotomy.

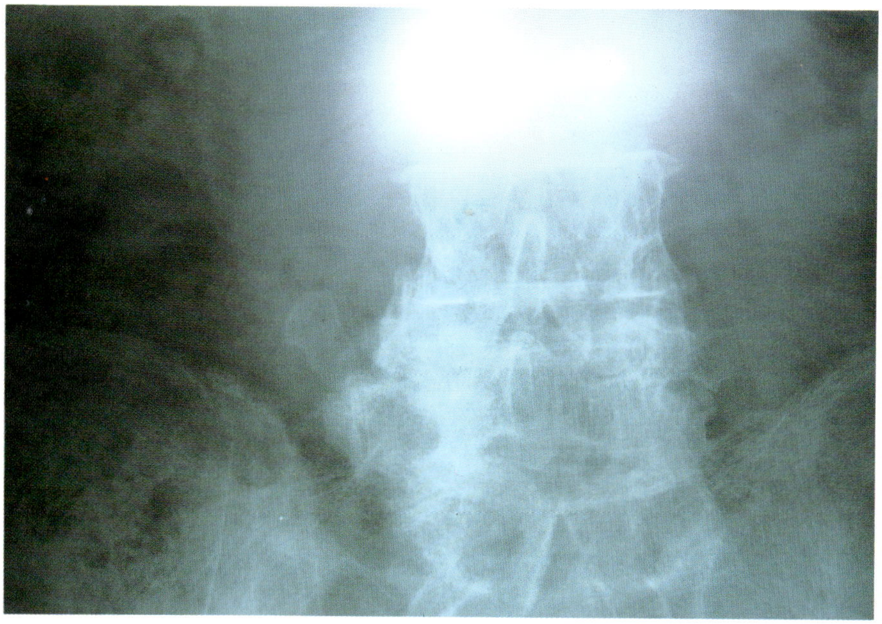

Fig. 14.4 An x-ray showing a middle third uretic stone recalcitrant to treatment by ESWL and ureteroscopy. This stone is suitable for a laparoscopic ureterolithotomy.

The 10mm or 12mm ports in the midclavicular and midaxillary lines facilitate the use of either the Babcock forceps or Endoclip Applier. Their adjacent 5mm ports are used for smaller manipulative and dissecting instruments (Fig. 14.2f).

Specific techniques

Ureterolysis

1 Dissection must proceed carefully and the positioning of an indwelling ureteric stent is essential. It can take some little time to discover the ureter and once this is achieved, a sling should be placed around it. This should not be brought out through one of the ports because there tends to be a continual gas leak. An (0) silk or Ethylon suture on a straight needle can be introduced percutaneously, taken around the ureter and then taken back out through the abdominal wall.

Dissection then continues until the whole of the ureter is free. An extra port may be required if the dissection goes across the pelvic brim. The freed ureter is then displaced laterally and it is fixed to the posterior abdominal wall either with interrupted sutures or with surgical clips.

2 A 5mm drain is inserted through one of the 5mm ports.

3 The ports are removed under direct vision and the wounds closed. A separate fascial suture will be necessary for 10mm wounds, but otherwise skin can be closed with either steristrips or a subcuticular suture. The ureteric stent should ideally be left in situ for at least two weeks.

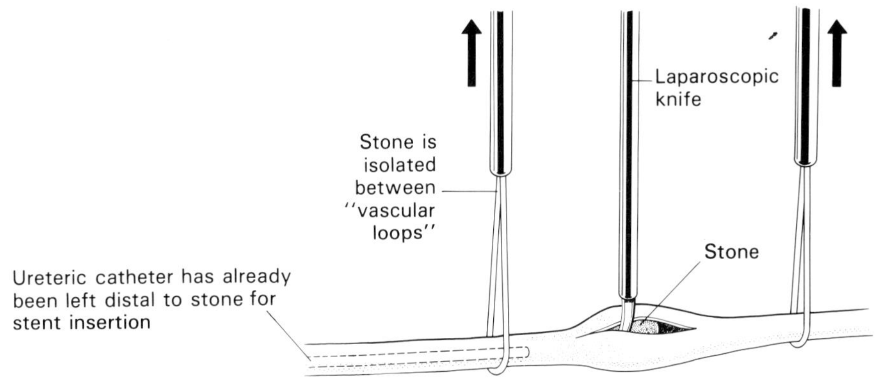

Fig. 14.5 Loops are placed around the ureter. The stone is delivered through a longitudinal incision that does not require suturing if a stent is pushed up from below.

Ureterolithotomy

1 The ureter should be identified within its sheath of periureteric fat at a point below the stone. There is usually a great deal of periureteric fibrosis around and above the site of an impacted stone and this is not the best place to start dissection. A sling is placed around the ureter (Fig. 14.5).
2 The ureter is then dissected to a point approximately 2cm above the stone and here a second sling is placed around the ureter.
3 The ureter is incised longitudinally over the stone (Fig. 14.5) and the stone lifted free and removed through one of the 10mm ports. A larger stone will require either enlargement of one of the port incisions subsequently or, as we prefer, placement within a small retrieval bag so that the stone can be safely squeezed through one of the 10mm ports without fear of the stone crumbling and dissemination of potential bacterial infection.
4 Suturing of the ureter is difficult and usually unnecessary. Stenting of the ureter is preferred and this can be carried out through the ureteric catheter that has already been left below the stone (Fig. 14.6).
5 A 5mm drain is inserted through one of the 5mm ports.
6 The ports are removed under direct vision and the wounds closed. A separate fascial suture will be necessary for 10mm wounds but otherwise skin can be closed with either steristrips or a subcuticular suture. The ureteric stent should ideally be left in situ for at least two weeks.

Nephrectomy

1 The ureter is identified above the pelvic brim, and the periureteric sheath is incised so that a sling can be placed around the ureter. It is easier to identify the ureter first, rather than dissect through the bulk of perinephric fat with the small laparoscopic scissors.

The ureter is followed up towards the hilum of the kidney. The kidney is then easily identified and the laparoscopic Babcock forceps

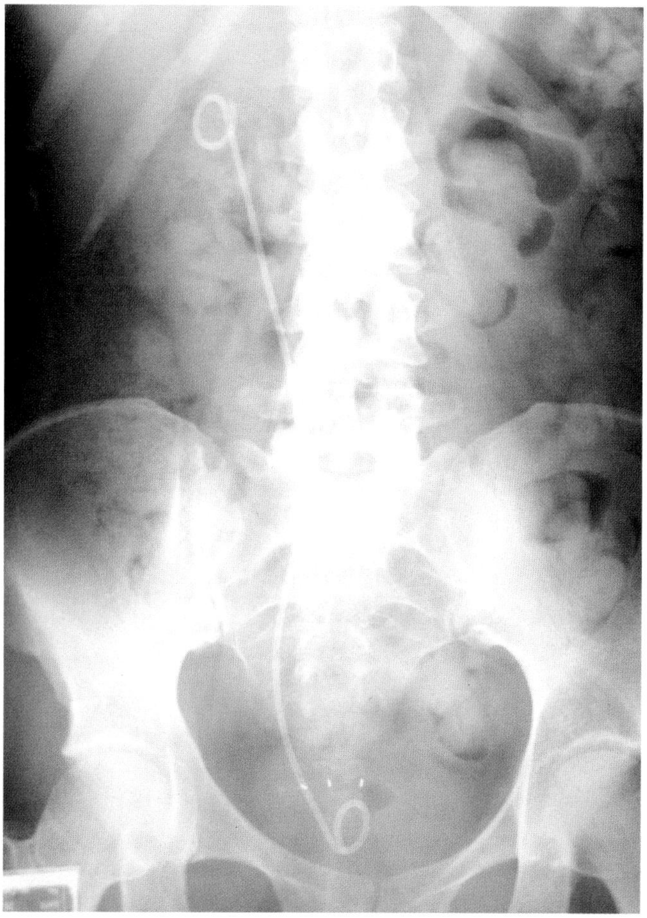

Fig. 14.6 A double pigtail stent is placed across the site of a laparoscopic ureterolithotomy, reducing the need for prolonged retroperitoneal drainage.

can be used to provide lateral retraction of the kidney by holding the renal pelvis.

2 The renal pedicle is then dissected with curved scissors and curved dissecting forceps until the individual vessels can accept either clips if they are less than 5 mm in diameter, or the Endo GIA 30 stapler if the vessels are larger (as in Fig. 15.6).

The artery should be clipped first although it is very tempting to take the more anteriorly placed vein before it. If the vein is obscuring the view of the artery, the vein can be gently pulled to one side with a silk loop.

3 A retrieval bag should be inserted through the 12 mm port in the midaxillary line. It should be taken down towards the pelvis and opened by insertion of the telescope. The opened neck should be held with grasping forceps and the kidney should be brought down into the bag using the Babcock forceps through the anterior 12 mm port (with spacer).

4 The neck of the bag is then brought out through the lateral 12 mm port and the kidney is morcellated using blunt Mayo scissors (Fig. 15.9). Fragments can be further broken down with the introduction of a finger and then removed with sponge-holding forceps. This must be visualized from within the retroperitoneal space to ensure that inadvertent perforation of the bag does not occur.

5 Close inspection is made of the renal bed, if necessary with irrigation and suction, to identify any further bleeding points. A 10mm drain is guided down under direct vision into the renal bed.

6 All ports are removed under direct vision.

7 The 10mm and 12mm wounds receive a fascial suture but otherwise all skin wounds only require steristrips or a subcuticular Dexon suture. The patient, who can usually tolerate an oral diet on the first postoperative day, can return home either on the first or second postoperative day. Normal activities can usually be resumed after about 10 days.

Pyeloplasty

1 The ureter is identified below the kidney and a loop is placed around the ureter and held up to the abdominal wall after incision through the periureteric sheath.

2 The ureter is dissected up to the renal pelvis. Some dissection of the lower pole of the kidney will be required to allow more lateral displacement of the kidney.

3 A holding suture should be placed either side of the stenotic segment. A third holding suture should be placed at the apex of the intended pyeloplasty (Fig. 14.7). These should be of 2/0 vicryl or Polysorb sutures because the colour is easy to see and the braided material is easier to knot laparoscopically.

4 The stenosed segment and the redundant pelvis are excised with scissors.

5 The reanastomosis is performed with two continuous 3/0 vicryl or Polysorb sutures (Fig. 14.8), one anteriorly and one posteriorly. The continuous sutures can be started and completed either with placement of a clip or with a knot.

6 Before completion of the anterior suture line, a guide-wire should be passed through the indwelling ureteric catheter up into the kidney for subsequent introduction of a double pigtail stent.

7 A 5mm wound drain is then guided down to the site of the pyeloplasty.

8 All ports are removed under direct vision and the carbon dioxide evacuated.

9 The 10mm and 12mm wounds receive a fascial suture, but otherwise all skin wounds require only steristrips or a subcuticular Dexon suture.

The drain can be removed on the first or second postoperative day in the absence of a urinary leak. The double pigtail stent should be removed after two weeks. The patient can usually tolerate an oral diet on the first postoperative day and returns home either on the first

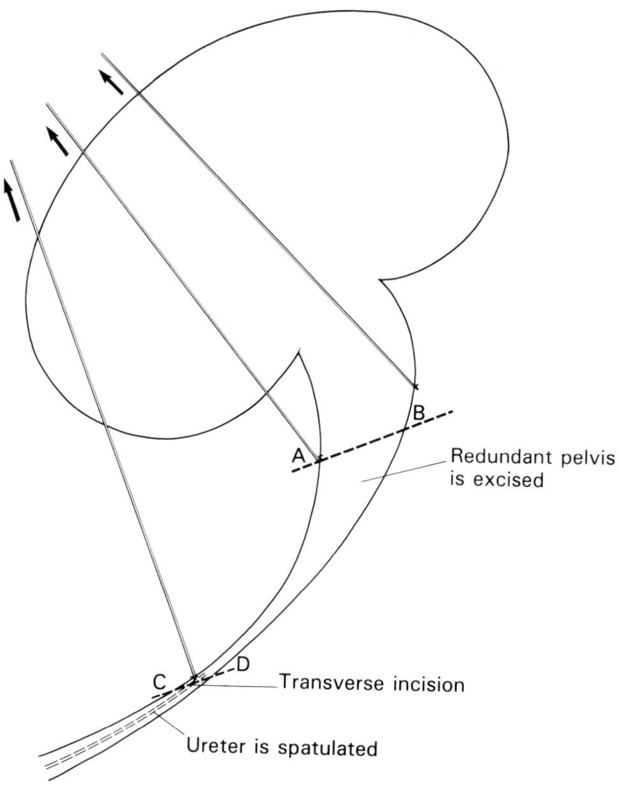

Fig. 14.7 Three holding sutures are placed prior to a laparoscopic pyeloplasty.

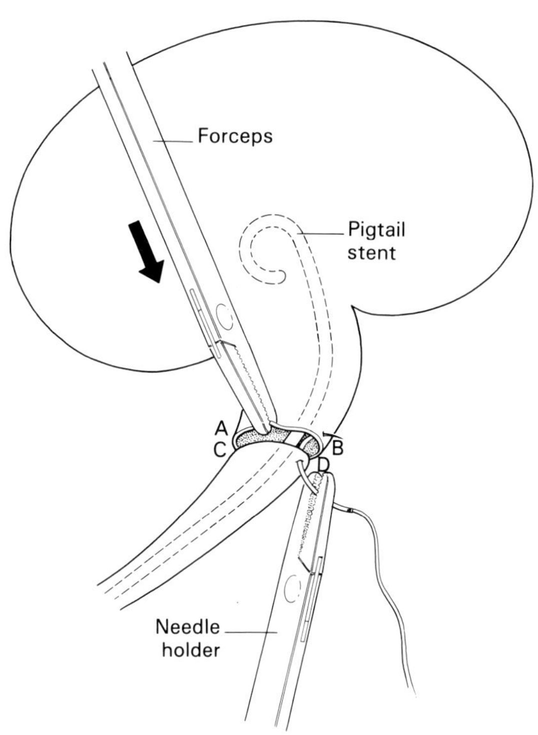

Fig. 14.8 The pyeloplasty is performed with two continuous 3/0 vicryl sutures.

or second postoperative day. Normal activities can be resumed after 10 days.

Discussion

At the present time, there is very little experience with retroperitoneal endoscopy. The greatest experience is with a ureterolithotomy (Gaur 1992, Lipskey & Wuernschinnel 1993). All of the cases reported have been successful and our own King's College Hospital experience is that this is an easily learned and rapid technique. Deroofment of a renal cyst (Morgan & Rader 1992) and a uretero-ureterostomy (Nezhat *et al.* 1992) have also been described.

There have been no reported complications with the ureterolithotomy, but we have found a persistent urinary leak through the drain occurs unless a double pigtail stent is placed across the site of the stone. This mirrors the experience with an open ureterolithotomy, but it has become more pertinent to reduce the duration of the urinary leak in a patient who could otherwise have been discharged from hospital because of the minimally invasive procedure.

The limiting factor for retroperitoneal endoscopy had been a lack of adequate working space. It has now become clear that the peritoneum can be peeled away with ease when a high pressure balloon is used. Pressures of up to 100 mmHg might induce a transient caval obstruction, but this has not yet been apparent. The anatomical restrictions are not yet documented, but in practice the space seems very crowded with ports and instruments. Only a small dysplastic kidney is at present suitable for a laparoscopic retroperitoneal nephrectomy.

Perinephric adhesions, whilst also a relative contraindication for a laparoscopic transperitoneal nephrectomy, make retroperitoneal insufflation dangerous, with the possible formation of a tension pneumoperitoneum if the peritoneum ruptures.

The laparoscopic pyeloplasty is an example of the feasibility of laparoscopy to copy an open dismembered pyeloplasty. We now await the assessment of alternative techniques such as laser soldering to fully exploit not only minimally invasive access but also precise endoscopic microsurgical dissection and manipulation.

References

Gaur D.D. (1992) Laparoscopic operative retroperitoneoscopy: Use of a new device. *Journal of Urology*, **148**, 1137–9.

Lipskey H. & Wuernschinnel E. (1993) Laparoscopic lithotomy for ureteral stones. *Minimally Invasive Therapy*, **2**: 1, 19–22.

Morgan C. & Rader D. (1992) Laparoscopic unroofing of a renal cyst. *Journal of Urology*, **148**, 1835–6.

Nezhat C., Nezhat F., Green B. (1992) Laparoscopic treatment of obstructed ureter due to endometriosis by resection and ??ureterureterostomy: A case report. *Journal of Urology*, **148**, 865–8.

Wickham J.E.A. & Miller R.A. (1983) Percutaneous renal access. In *Percutaneous renal surgery* (J.E.A. Wickham & R.A. Miller), pp. 33–9. Churchill Livingstone, New York.

15: Laparoscopic Transperitoneal Nephrectomy

M. J. COPTCOAT AND A. D. JOYCE

Introduction

There was great excitement at the 1991 meeting of the American Urological Association in Toronto when Ralph Clayman presented his series of four patients who had undergone a laparoscopic nephrectomy. His series has increased (Clayman *et al.* 1991) as have those from other centres around the world.

Clayman introduced the concept of dissecting the kidney laparoscopically through the peritoneal space, delivering the organ into an impermeable bag, bringing the bag neck out of the abdomen and inserting a morcellating device to remove the tissue. It is his application of the bag principle that has made this operation safe and feasible. Rassweiler and Coptcoat carried out laparoscopic nephrectomies in dogs in 1990, removing the kidneys with the endoscopic liquidizer and surgical aspirator (ELSA). However, both these cases required initial embolization and the subsequent tissue removal was haphazard, difficult to visualize and deemed to be dangerous. Thus, the use of an impermeable bag to protect other organs and to allow safe, blind liquidization or morcellation is an advance.

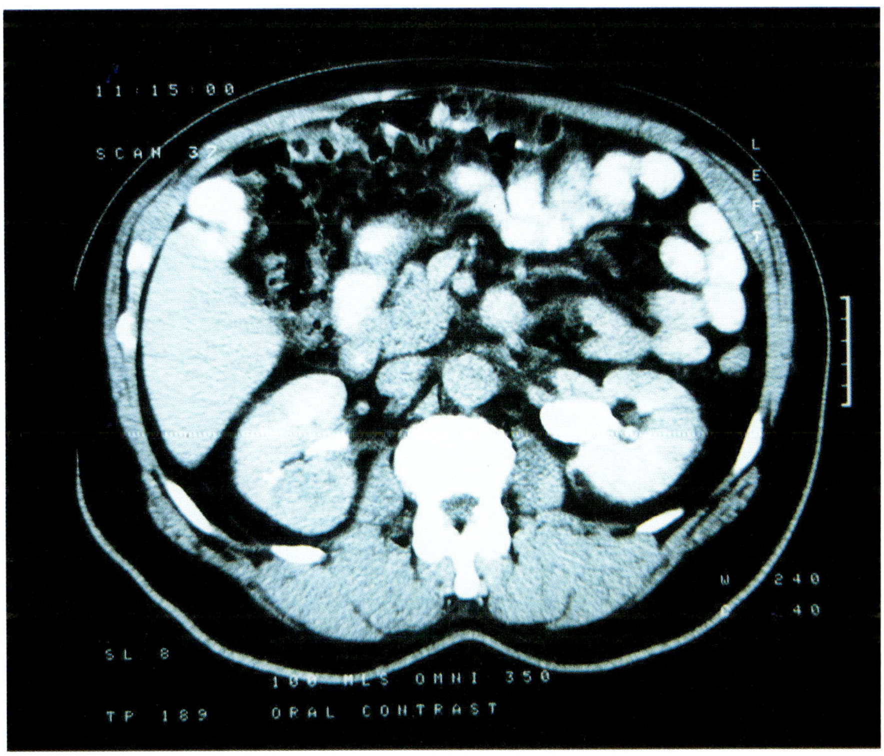

Fig 15.1 A CT scan of a small renal cell cancer suitable for a laparoscopic 'radical' transperitoneal radical nephrectomy.

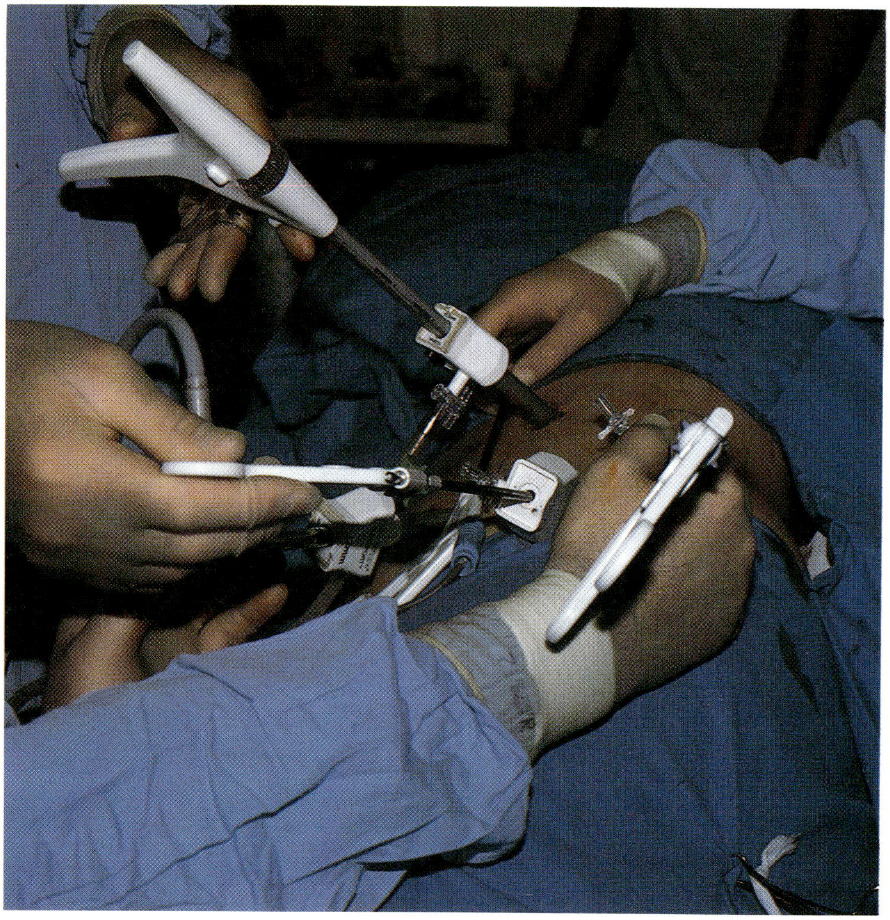

Fig 15.2 An overview of the ports used for a laparoscopic transperitoneal nephrectomy. The Veress needle was inserted at the site for the telescope.

An open nephrectomy for either benign or malignant renal pathology is not usually a technically difficult procedure, but is associated with a 10% incidence of incisional complications, a 10% incidence of chest infections and a mortality rate of 1.4%. The hospital stay after an open nephrectomy averages 6–10 days, even amongst the healthiest patients who are donating a kidney for transplantation (De Marco *et al.* 1982).

It is the trauma and morbidity associated with the access through the abdominal musculature that has prompted many of us to consider a laparoscopic version. We now have experience with over 47 cases of laparoscopic nephrectomy and nephroureterectomy between our two departments. The initial success of the laparoscopic nephrectomy for benign disease and subsequent evaluation of the impermeable bags made of Ripstop balloon nylon led us to undertake a laparoscopic nephrectomy for malignant renal pathology (Fig. 15.1).

When one witnesses a patient being able to take an oral diet within 24 hours of a laparoscopic radical nephrectomy, go home within three or four days and return to normal activities at a mean time of 29 days, one is witnessing all of the hallmarks of a truly minimally invasive procedure that can now be applied to cancer surgery.

Laparoscopic instrumentation

Simple nephrectomy

1 High-flow carbon dioxide insufflator
2 CCD camera and two monitors
3 Veress needle (safety type)
4 0° 10mm laparoscope (30° optional)
5 Two 10mm ports with grips and converters/two 5mm downsizers
6 Two 12mm ports with grips and converters/two 10mm, two 5mm downsizers
7 Laparoscopic scissors (diathermy connection)
8 Laparoscopic dissecting forceps
9 Laparoscopic Babcock grasping forceps
10 Laparoscopic soft grasping forceps
11 Endoclip* Applier (medium/large)
12 Endo GIA* 30 stapler
13 Entrapment/retrieval bag
14 Fan retractor

Radical nephrectomy and nephroureterectomy

As for a simple nephrectomy, with the addition of one to two 5mm ports with grips.

Techniques

General technique for nephrectomy

1 Under a general anaesthetic with muscle paralysis and assisted ventilation, the patient is put into a lateral position with the table broken between the ribs and iliac crest (as in Fig. 14.1). The layout of equipment is shown in Chapter 13 (Fig. 13.2)

The patient can be held by straps or preferably supported on a rest with slight backward tilt. A urethral catheter is required but ureteric intubation is not. Thrombo-embolic deterrent stockings are recommended.

2 The Veress needle is inserted horizontally at the edge of the rectus sheath in line with the umbilicus and will also be the site for the telescope port (Fig. 15.2). A long needle is require for all but the thinnest patients. The infusion and drop tests are performed. Early insufflation is often prevented by a high intra-abdominal pressure (over 12mmHg) feedback, but this is usually due to malpositioning of the needle tip. It is countered by gently lifting the tip up laterally

*A trademark of the United States Surgical Corporation (AutoSuture).

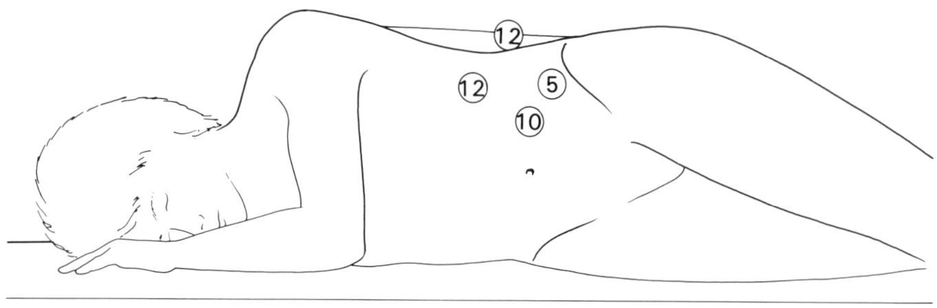

Fig. 15.3 The port sites for a laparoscopic transperitoneal nephrectomy.

where it becomes free from the colon. Insufflate 2–4 litres of carbon dioxide.

3 The Veress needle is removed. The skin incision is lengthened horizontally to 11 mm and a disposable 10mm port with grip inserted (Fig. 15.3). The carbon dioxide is connected to this port until secondary ports have been added.

4 Inspect the abdomen with the laparoscope. Identify the potential sites for secondary ports which should be well away from superficial vessels.

Insert two secondary ports under direct vision in the midclavicular line. These ports are the principal sites for the dissection instruments used by the operator. Keep the 12mm port, which is for the Endo GIA 30 stapler, at least 2cm below the ribs to allow greater freedom of movement.

A short interchange of telescope with the larger secondary port will allow visual adjustment of the grip and cannula of the first telescope port. Subsequent carbon dioxide insufflation should be through a secondary port to prevent unnecessary local cooling of the telescope. The telescope should be prewarmed to body core temperature.

5 The peritoneal reflection lateral to the colon is incised from the hepatic or splenic flexure down to the pelvic brim (Fig. 15.4). The use of the lateral position facilitates medial displacement of the colon by virtue of gravity. A mild preoperative phosphate enema will also have helped reduce the bulk of the colon.

Although this plane is said to be bloodless, there is often a small artery at either end of the reflection. These, together with the usually trivial superficial peritoneal vessels which require diathermy haemostasis to prevent small haemorrhages accumulatively absorb the light. Such oozing is precipitated by vasodilatation caused by local carbon dioxide absorption but is never so severe as to be anything other than a nuisance for camera visualization. The problem of fading light due to haemoglobin absorption can be easily countered by inserting an unfolded white swab and using this for background reflection.

6 A single 12mm port can then be safely placed in the midaxillary line to be used for ureteric and renal retraction and bag introduction. A fifth port (5mm) may be necessary in the midaxillary line if extra

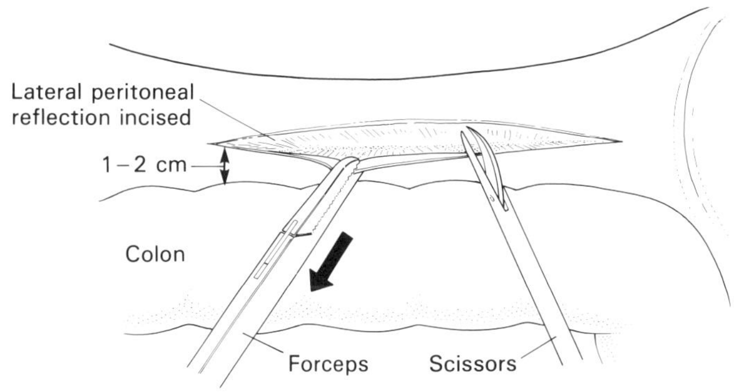

Fig. 15.4 The peritoneal reflection lateral to the colon is incised from the hepatic or splenic flexure down to the pelvic brim at the beginning of a laparoscopic transperitoneal nephrectomy.

retraction is required, particularly to separate the liver from the upper pole of the right kidney.

7 The next step is identification, clipping, division and retraction of the proximal ureter (Fig. 15.5). It is most easily found at the pelvic brim as it runs over the iliac vessels. This is the same manoeuvre for dissection of both benign and malignant renal pathologies.

The ureter can be followed up to the kidney with gradually higher retraction using Babcock forceps through a lateral port. The gonadal vein can either be bypassed or clipped and divided where it crosses the ureter. A hydronephrotic kidney is best aspirated at this stage to make subsequent manipulation and ultimate removal easier.

8 The perinephric fat is incised. The renal pedicle is displayed by lateral traction of the kidney and gentle shearing of soft tissues at the hilum with partially open laparoscopic scissors. This results in a well dissected pedicle that can be separated by a loop and is ready for clipping (Fig. 15.6). The vessels are clipped if less than 5 mm in diameter. Clean dissection is required to produce a snug fit of the clips. Larger vessels require the Endo GIA 30 stapler. This instrument places six 3 mm rows of staples across each vessel and incises between them. The artery and vein should not be included at the same time, except as a last resort because of the risk of arterio-venous fistula formation.

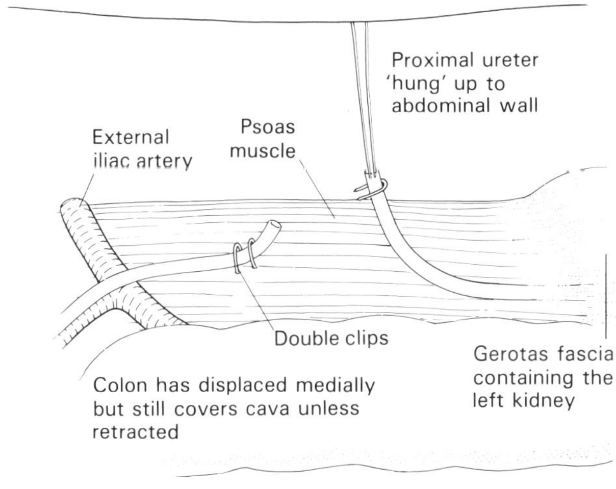

Fig. 15.5 The ureter is identified, clipped and divided as it passes over the pelvic brim. The proximal end can be held up with a suture to the abdominal wall. Dissection then proceeds along the ureter up to the kidney.

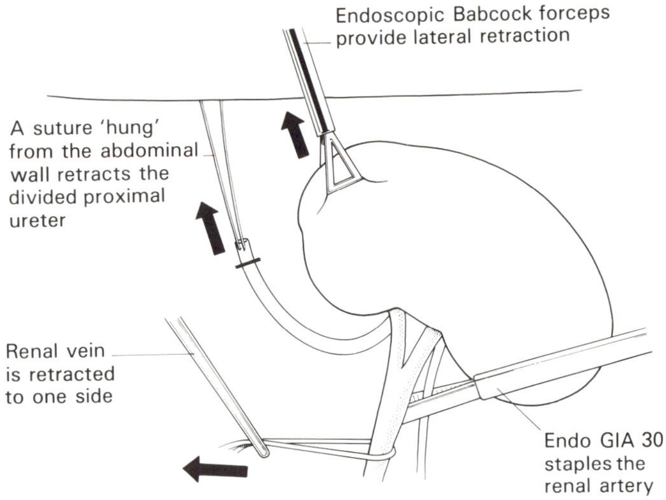

Fig. 15.6 The renal pedicle is displayed by lateral traction of the kidney and the gentle shearing effect on the soft tissues at the hilum with partially open laparoscopic scissors. The renal vein is pulled to one side with a small tape or ligature, giving enough room for the Endo GIA 30 stapler to secure and incise the renal artery.

Do not be tempted to clip the vessels too close to the kidney because it is then common to find that you have only secured a branch rather than the main vessel itself.

9 The freed kidney should be put in a specially designed organ entrapment bag. The bag is inserted through a 12mm port laterally and placed in the pelvis away from the kidney (Fig. 15.7). The telescope is

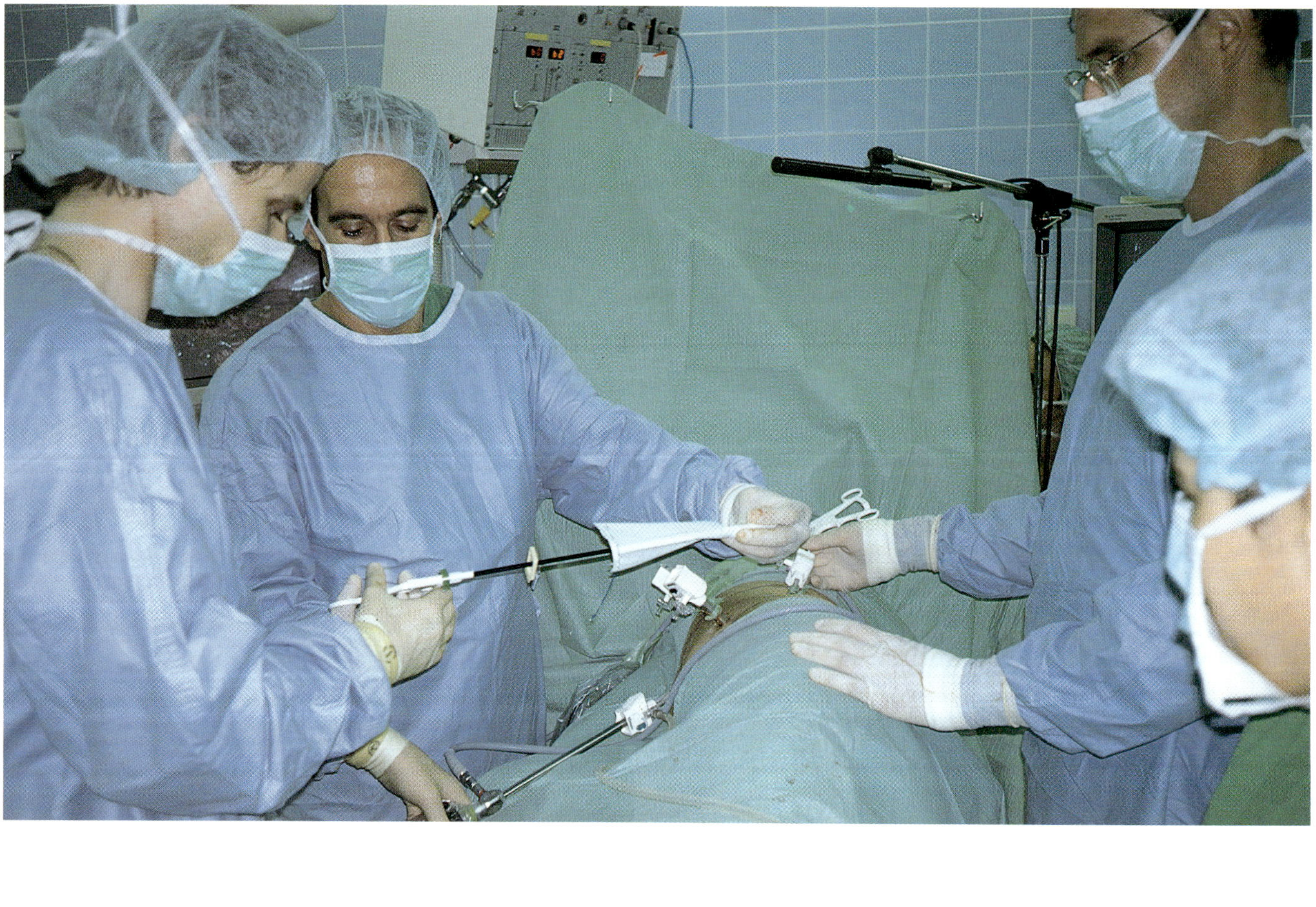

Fig. 15.7 The organ retrieval bag is inserted through a lateral 12mm port and placed in the pelvis.

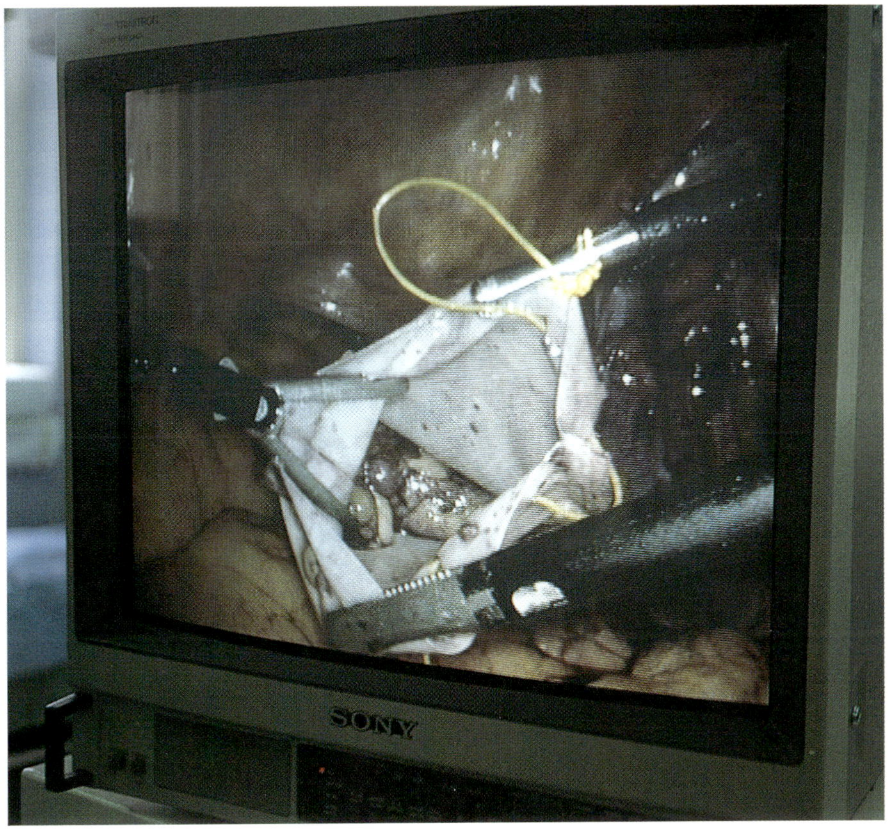

Fig 15.8 The dissected kidney is placed in an organ retrieval bag.

pushed into the neck and a gentle rotating movement will unravel and open the sac fully. Two pairs of forceps are required for holding open the sac and the Babcock forceps can then be used to swing the kidney down into the bag (Fig. 15.8). The shape of the impermeable bag made of coated nylon facilitates both easy entrapment and a neck closure on removal.

10 The neck of the bag is brought out through the lateral 12mm port site. The renal bed is inspected, irrigated and aspirated to check for haemorrhage. This can be difficult to detect beneath a blood clot and meticulous inspection is recommended with gauze swabbing if necessary to prevent the frustration of bringing a patient back to theatre for an accumulating haemorrhage from a minor origin.

11 The bag should be visualized throughout morcellation to identify any possible entrapment of the sac with whatever morcellating dcvicc is uscd. Thc simplcst and safcst morccllation tcchniquc has been the fragmentation of the kidney by a combination of blunt-nosed Mayo scissors and finger manipulation (the incision may need to be enlarged to 2cm). The fragments are then removed with sponge-holding forceps (Fig. 15.9).

12 A drain is placed through one of the 5mm port sites to facilitate rapid removal of carbon dioxide and provide an indicator for possible haemorrhage. It can be removed on the first postoperative day.

13 A fascial suture is required for10mm and 12mm puncture sites.

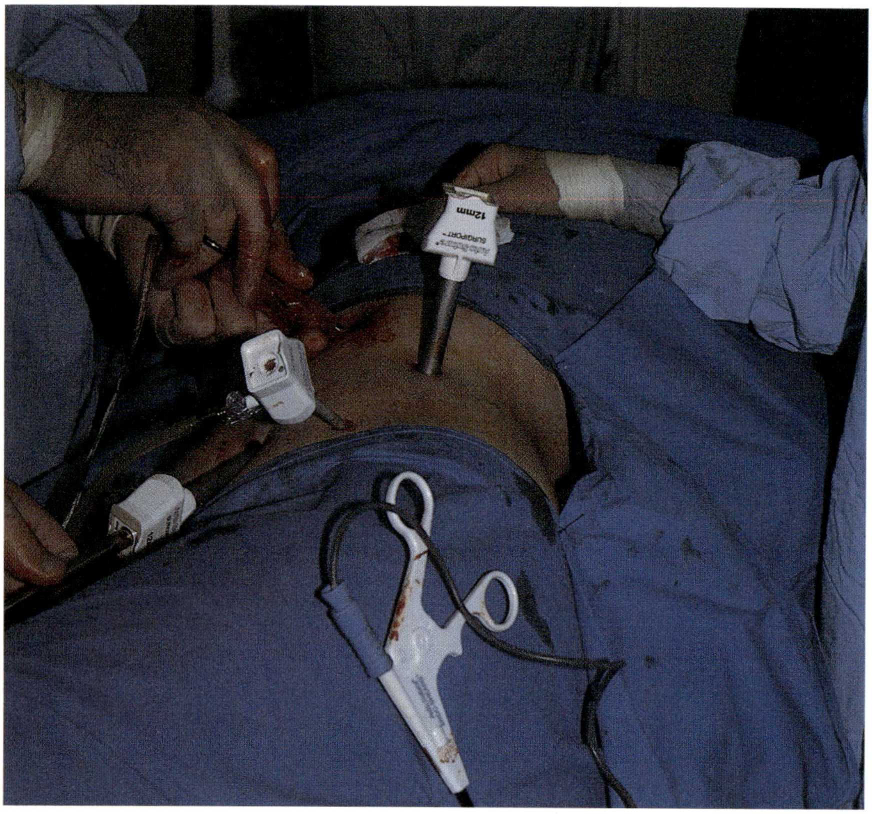

Fig. 15.9 The kidney is fragmented by a combination of scissor and finger morcellation through the neck of the bag. The fragments are then removed with sponge-holding forceps.

Steristrips are suitable for some female patients but generally more active patients are best given a simple 3/0 Ethylon suture to each skin wound.

General technique for nephroureterectomy

For benign pathology such as reflux nephropathy

An extra 5 mm port should be inserted at the edge of the rectus sheath in line with the anterior superior iliac spine (Fig. 5.10). The distal end of the ureter can then be dissected downwards until the bladder is reached. It is usually possible to get a 10mm clip across the ureter at least 1–2 cm away from the bladder. If there is a megaureter which requires division, the extra port should be of a 12 mm size so that the Endo GIA 30 stapler can easily be placed deep into the pelvis to run across the ureter as close as possible to the bladder. A urethral catheter is left in situ for three days.

For renal transitional cell cancer

Because of the possibility of leaving a small ureteric stump, we prefer to circumcise the ureteric orifice transurethrally with a diathermy knife before the laparoscopic procedure begins. Subsequent dissection

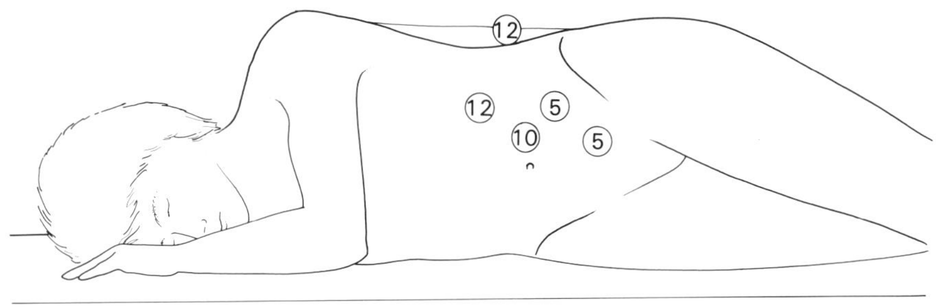

Fig 15.10 The ports used for a laparoscopic transperitoneal nephroureterectomy. An additional 5cm port is placed in the pelvis.

as described immediately above down towards the bladder will then facilitate easy removal of the whole ureter from the bladder. A urethral catheter should be left in situ for approximately 10 days until bladder healing occurs.

Results

Benign pathology

Out of 40 patients 38 underwent a successful laparoscopic nephrectomy with a mean operating time of 2.5 hours (range 1.3–6.5). However, two of the 38 completed cases required an open exploration four and six hours later for suspected haemorrhage.

One patient was found to have a 4mm tear in the stump of the renal vein. The second case was slowly leaking from a missed suprarenal arterial branch. A third patient who developed a secondary haemorrhage 18 hours postoperatively was successfully managed conservatively. These three cases were the only ones to require blood transfusions. Both the cases that were abandoned peroperatively had densely adherent kidneys containing staghorn stones and previous histories of a perinephric abscess. Laparoscopic dissection seemed to be making little progress and these cases were converted to an open nephrectomy.

Thus the overall success in avoiding an open procedure in this group was 36 out of 40 (90%). The patients had no wound or respiratory complications.

One patient experienced several peroperative and postoperative cardiac dysrhythmias due to a persistent metabolic acidosis that could not be compensated for by assisted ventilation. This had been one of the longer earlier cases (5.5 hours). There have been no other complications.

The mean in-patient stay was three days (range 2–7) and the mean return to normal activities was 10.7 days (range 2–21). The mean operating time was 1.5 hours for a dysplastic kidney, 2.3 hours for a hydronephrotic kidney and 3.2 hours to complete a nephroureterectomy for reflux nephropathy.

Renal cancer

All seven patients underwent a successful laparoscopic nephrectomy with a mean operating time of 3.5 hours (range 2.5–5.0). There were no preoperative or postoperative complications and no blood transfusions were required. The mean in-patient stay was 5.2 days (range 3–9) and the mean return to normal activities was 29 days (range 18–36). The two patients who had undergone a laparoscopic nephroureterectomy were discharged home with a urethral catheter which was left in situ for 10 days.

In the cases of renal cell cancer, histopathological assessment of the fragmented tissue specimens confirmed the preoperative diagnosis and did not show any involvement of fat or lymph-node tissue. In one of the renal transitional cell carcinomas (poorly differentiated), involvement of lymphatics was noted. This patient developed para-aortic nodal metastases and tumour in the renal bed eight months postoperatively and died after developing pulmonary metastases. The patients were followed up for a mean of 14.7 months (range 11–19 months) and this is the only recurrence identified on follow-up CT scanning.

Discussion

Both the laparoscopic nephrectomy and laparoscopic radical nephrectomy have proved to be safe and effective techniques, avoiding the morbidity associated with an open nephrectomy. Our technique has gradually been refined over the 47 cases, and our indications for a laparoscopic nephrectomy now include dysplasia, reflux nephropathy, hydronephrosis, stage 1 renal cell cancer, transitional cell cancer and other intrarenal lesions.

Contraindications

The possibility of dense perirenal fibrosis in patients with a history of a perinephric abscess or previous open surgery (previous percutaneous surgery has not been a problem in two of our cases) are at present relative contraindications. An absolute contraindication should be renal tumours that breach the capsule or invade the renal vein. This point reinforces the need for accurate preoperative staging with CT and venography if indicated. An arteriogram is not essential for diagnosis and staging, but it provides valuable anatomical orientation when undertaking a laparoscopic radical nephrectomy for cancer.

Laparoscopically assisted nephrectomy

The size of the tumour is important. The mass of a normal kidney with up to a 5 cm tumour can be managed entirely laparoscopically. Larger tumours can still be removed in a minimally invasive way but with the assistance of a hand placed in the abdomen through a distant Lanz-type incision, from which the specimen can be removed intact. Contrary to the philosophy of reducing the trauma of access, this compromise will increase the indication of this and other laparoscopic operations and enable a better final check of haemostasis.

Laparoscopy for renal cancer

The initial success of the laparoscopic nephrectomy for benign disease and the subsequent improvement in the design of organ entrapment bags has allowed us to extend the indications of the minimally invasive technique to renal cancer. It is much easier laparoscopically to dissect around the perinephric fat of a kidney containing a renal tumour than it is to dissect through the fat of a previously infected kidney.

This lends itself to facilitation of a radical dissection and is combined with following the plane of the great vessels upwards to ensure inclusion of hilar nodes. The disadvantage is that a much larger specimen is dissected, which has required much larger organ bags and greater team skills in placement of the specimen into the bag with minimal manipulation.

An early step of any open nephrectomy for renal cell cancer is control of the renal vein to reduce the possibility of embolization. The technique of laparoscopic dissection that has been described above starts with the pelvic ureter. This has been found to be an advantage in that the pedicle is reached, although indirectly, with greater certainty and less unnecessary dissection through incorrect tissue planes. The possibility of venous tumour embolization is also probably reduced by the minimal manipulation of the kidney which occurs in laparoscopic surgery.

A silk (0) sling can usually be placed around the renal vein to reduce further the likelihood of embolization and also to facilitate better access of the Endo GIA 30 stapler to the renal artery which must be taken first. The principle of minimal handling also applies to manipulation of the bowel and minimal handling may explain why any postoperative ileus is so short when compared to that following open nephrectomy.

The organ entrapment bag

Once the specimen is trapped within the organ bag, the neck is pulled out of the abdomen. This isolates the specimen from the peritoneal cavity, but impermeability is essential to avoid potential seeding of malignant cells as the tissue is fragmented. Our bags, designed by

Harry Espiner, a general surgeon from Bristol, England, have been rigorously tested to exclude this possibility. The bags have a Wesoloski porosity index of less than 50 mm/cm^2/minute under test conditions using serum.

Electron microscopy evaluation has failed to demonstrate leakage of any cells through the bags, even under high pressure. The development of metastatic tumour in the patient with poorly differentiated transitional cell carcinoma was almost certainly a reflection of established microscopic lymphatic spread, as suggested by the histological assessment of the nephrectomy specimen. Such cases are uncommon and they always have a poor prognosis. Preoperatively, it would have been impossible to stage this patient correctly. We concluded that seeding of the tumour did not occur through the retrieval bag during morcellation.

Organ entrapment bags or retrieval devices are in essence simple impermeable bags which are used to collect a variety of organs and tissues within the abdomen and bring them safely onto the abdominal wall via one of the ports. They were first introduced for infected or 'hot' gallbladders but are now used for the removal of bowel tumours and end organs such as the ovary, kidney and spleen. They are much more than just a bag in that they must be of such a design to be easily introduced through a port and be strong enough to withstand the morcellatión that is required when the tissue is too bulky to bring out directly through the abdominal wall. Once the neck of the bag has been brought out to the surface, then any further dissection or morcellation becomes extracorporeal and there is no danger of seeding possible tumour cells back into the peritoneum.

Much credit in this area must go to Ralph Clayman who used the idea of a bag to assist in the removal of a kidney during a laparoscopic nephrectomy (Clayman *et al.* 1990). Until then, many people had looked upon the possibility of a laparoscopic nephrectomy in a very sceptical way since morcellation within the abdomen could only be dangerous when not protected by a bag.

Tissue morcellation

Morcellation devices are required when the tissue bulk is greater than the diameter of the port or lip of the sack. There is a variety of crude devices available, and we will surely see a great refinement of these in the near future.

The main problem is the morcellation and removal of fibrous connective tissue, which tends to obstruct both the cutting and aspirating channels of these instruments. At present, there does not seem to be very much difference between inserting a pair of blunt-nosed Mayo scissors and fragmenting the tissue and employing the electrical devices which either liquidize or morcellate the tissue.

One of the disadvantages of morcellating tissue is that accurate staging of a possible tumour by the histopathologist is very difficult, if not sometimes impossible. This means that preoperative staging must be as thorough as possible, and in the case of renal tumours CT scanning is essential in every case, when previously one might have operated solely with an IVU (intravenous urogram) and ultrasound. However, the type of tissue and possible tumour can be identified even with liquidized samples and this also lends itself to DNA analysis using flow cytometry.

Examples of existing endoscopic tissue removal techniques include scissor/forcep combinations and tissue compression in laparoscopy, rotating side cutters in arthroscopy and diathermy cutting loops in urology.

More experimental is the application of alternative sources of energy to disrupt tissue; both light and sound energy have been tried. Some lasers are effective in vaporizing tissue but these are generally not of the right wavelength to pass down an optical fibre. Lasers that are currently suitable for endoscopic application such as the Nd:YAG laser require too much power and generate high temperatures when used for tissue vaporization and cannot be used for large scale tissue destruction. Ultrasonic tissue removal has been used at open operation and endoscopically; although good at removing cellular material, it leaves behind fibrous tissue and its power is limited when applied through an endoscope. A motor-driven probe has been described that overcomes some of the limitations of ultrasound generation, particularly the length of the instrument, but no clinical application was reported (Coptcoat *et al.* 1988).

The endoscopic liquidizer and surgical aspirator (ELSA) was developed at the Institute of Urology primarily as a device to remove prostatic tissue endoscopically, but larger devices were also made to be used laparoscopically. The ELSA has been described elsewhere and has been used successfully to remove a variety of tissues in urological procedures such as benign prostatic hyperplasia, superficial bladder tumours and ovarian and uterine tissue at laparoscopy (Coptcoat *et al.* 1988). The ELSA was used during our first laparoscopic nephrectomy cases but it too became obstructed with the fibrous tissue from the pelvicalyceal system, and we now find that the simple use of Mayo scissors for fragmentation and of sponge holding forceps for tissue removal to be just as efficient.

Clayman has described an automatic punch (Clayman *et al.* 1990) which aspirates the cut tissue into a reservoir. This was used successfully in his early pig experiments and has proved to be an efficient tool in his current clinical series of laparoscopic nephrectomies, although it also sometimes becomes obstructed with fibrous tissue (personal communication). Unfortunately, this instrument is not available at the time of writing, and so alternative low-tech methods are being employed by other urologists such as ourselves. This continues to be an area of research in many centres and it will not be long before new, exciting, efficient and safe devices are available.

The exact technique for removing tissue from an organ bag to facilitate removal of an organ through a 1 cm incision is still being evaluated. There are hi-tech automated morcellating devices in use clinically but at the present time, the process can still be efficiently undertaken with a pair of blunt-nosed scissors, a finger and sponge-holding forceps. The tissue is incised, fragmented with the finger and withdrawn with the forceps.

Morcellated tissue comprising 0.5–1 cm fragments allows the histopathologist to make a histological diagnosis of the tumour, extension into perinephric fat and nodes if present, but preoperative clinical staging by CT or MRI is mandatory. Extraction of the intact specimen through a small midline incision or per vagina in a female has been considered but excluded on the grounds of unnecessary trauma and invasiveness.

Much of the argument concerning whether a laparoscopic nephrectomy is safe for renal cancer has centred on the theoretical possibility of tumour-cell seeding. I think that this argument has been logically countered and is backed up with the clinical series reported. However, there is a positive side to a laparoscopic technique for the removal of malignant renal pathology. This centres on the reduced handling and more refined dissection of tissues, together with a definite protection of the patient's immune system because of the reduced trauma of access, which may play an important part in the patient's resistance to seeding of metastatic tumour cells both during the operation and until the patient fully recovers.

Lundy *et al.* (1979) used a murine metastatic tumour system as a model to assess the effects of a major surgical procedure on tumour-specific immune reactivity and the growth of micrometastases. Any major surgical procedure carried out on these animals resulted in impaired cell-mediated cytotoxicity postoperatively and an increase in the number of gross pulmonary metastases when computed with minor procedures.

Horgan (Horgan *et al.* 1992) has shown in an animal model that a laparotomy produced significantly suppressed lymphocyte proliferation rates compared with a laparoscopy group. This experiment parallels the initial work of Lundy and now requires a series of experiments to compare the growth of micrometastases in animals which have undergone both laparoscopy and laparotomy.

Logic would predict that the least immuno-compromised laparoscopic group should develop far fewer metastases. This is one large but reasonable theoretical leap away from a clinical situation for human renal cancer and only follow-up of our series over the next 5–10 years may even suggest that this is pertinent.

Laparoscopic nephroureterectomy

Transitional cell cancer of the kidney or ureter requires a nephroureterectomy. The laparoscopic nephroureterectomy for benign reflux nephropathy is a straightforward operation, requiring an additional pelvic port, but subsequent cystograms have shown that a 1–2 cm ureteric stump is left when the dissection seems complete, probably because of the difficulty in getting either a clip or stapler right down onto the bladder. This is not a clinical problem, however, for these cases.

An alternative to the open two-incision nephroureterectomy has been described (Abercrombie 1972) where the intravesical portion of the ureter is initially circumcised with a transurethral endoscopic diathermy knife, allowing the ureter to be pulled up through the loin incision. This has proved to be an effective cancer operation on long-term follow-up (Abercrombie *et al.* 1988).

Our approach to a laparoscopic nephroureterectomy for cancer has been to adopt the same technique for release of the intravesical portion of the ureter, and there is no theoretical reason why the laparoscopic version should not also be safe. A urethral catheter with a balloon inflated to 10 ml should be pulled down onto the bladder neck to prevent CO_2 escape through the bladder during the subsequent laparoscopy. The ureter can be dissected laparoscopically down to the bladder through the same ports, pulled away from the bladder and included in the organ bag.

Operating time

A laparoscopic radical nephrectomy has a longer mean operating time than a laparoscopic nephrectomy in our series, as well as producing a slightly longer postoperative stay. This partly reflects the need for more precise dissection and conservative postoperative care in this subgroup, but it can also be explained by the older age-group concerned. However, the morbidity, in terms of chest and wound complications, is still much less than even the best candidates for an open nephrectomy, i.e. those undergoing a live donor transplant nephrectomy (De Marco *et al.* 1982).

The mean operating time for any type of laparoscopic nephrectomy has fallen dramatically. This does not just reflect our increasing experience with this specific procedure but also the increasing indications of laparoscopy in urology. The immediate horizon will reveal safe techniques for partial nephrectomy, possibly using laparoscopic doppler and ultrasound probes, but at present we believe that the pioneering work of Clayman has led to a safe, efficacious, minimally invasive technique that can be applied to both benign and malignant renal pathology.

References

Abercrombie G.F. (1972) Nephroureterectomy. *Proceedings of the Royal Society of Medicine*, **65**, 1021–2.

Abercrombie G.F., Eardley I., Payne S., Walmsley B.H., Vinnicombe J. (1988) Modified nephroureterectomy. Long-term follow-up with particular reference to subsequent bladder tumours. *British Journal of Urology*, **61**, 198–200.

Clayman R., Kavoussi L., Long S.R., Dierks S.M., Meretyk S., Soper N. (1990) Laparoscopic nephrectomy. Initial report of pelvioscopic organ ablation in the pig. *Journal of Endourology*, **4**, 247.

Clayman R., Kavoussi L., Soper N. *et al.* (1991) Laparoscopic nephrectomy: Initial case report. *Journal of Urology*, **146**, 278–82.

Coptcoat M.J., Ison K.T., Wickham J.E.A. (1988) Endoscopic tissue liquidization and surgical aspiration. *Journal of Endourology*, **2**, 321.

Coptcoat M.J. (1991) Endoscopic liqidisation of the kidney, bladder and prostate. ChM thesis. Liverpool University.

De Marco T., Amin M., Harty J. (1982) Living donor nephrectomy: factors influencing morbidity. *Journal of Urology*, **127**, 1082–3.

Horgan P.G., Fitzpatrick M., Couse N., Gorey T., Fitzpatrick J.M. (1992) Laparoscopy is less immuno-traumatic than laparotomy. *Minimally Invasive Therapy*, **1**, 241–4.

Lundy J., Lovett E., Wolinsky B., Conran P. (1979) Immune impairment and metastatic tumour growth. *Cancer*, **43**, 945–51.

16: Laparoscopic Colposuspension

M.J. COPTCOAT AND P. CARTER

Introduction

The prevalence of female urinary incontinence in the community remains between 7% and 12%, with approximately 75% of these cases being due to genuine stress incontinence (Krantz 1986). Over 100 different operations have been described using either a suprapubic, or transvaginal approach or a combination of both, but none as yet have proved to be a satisfactory procedure for all patients presenting with incontinence. The fundamental principle of performing the best operation first is undisputed, but considerable differences of opinion exist as to exactly which this operation may be.

The surgical options may be divided according to the approach, with the more complex procedures such as artificial sphincters, urinary diversion and injection techniques not further mentioned here.

Anterior colporrhaphy has the advantage of allowing correction of a cystocele or cystourethrocele at the same time as aiming to restore the bladder neck to its normal position with restoration of pressure transmission to the urethra (Weil *et al.* 1984). It is a short and relatively simple procedure which is performed transvaginally and aims to approximate the pubocervical fascia anterior to the urethra and so supporting the bladder neck. The complications of the procedure are infrequent but include damage to the bladder or urethra and local haematoma formation. Later problems include recurrent prolapse, urinary incontinence, dyspareunia and urethral stricture. Reported cure rates vary from 40–90% on subjective analysis but the long-term cure rate for incontinence is poor. With the possible exception of the elderly or frail, where operative morbidity may dictate the choice of surgery, anterior colporrhaphy is not felt to be the best option for isolated stress incontinence (Cardozo & Cutner 1992).

Endoscopic bladder-neck suspension was first described by Pereyra (1959) and subsequently modified by many authors (Cardozo 1992). In all procedures, the same principles of bladder-neck suspension from the anterior rectus sheath are employed, by means of nonabsorbable sutures through the paravesical tissues, with cystoscopic examination to ensure correct placement. Subjective cure rates, in the region of 90%, appear to be best from authors who describe the technique. However, objective results from some series are disappointing, with reported cure rates of 40% or less (Mundy 1983, Kirby & Whiteway 1989). The advantages of the procedure are its minimal operative morbidity, with a short in-patient stay, and particularly the option of using local anaesthetic. This makes it an attractive procedure for the frail and elderly, and its poor success rate in many series may well be due to the fact that it is reserved for such patients, whose tissues and healing powers are less than optimal. Complications are few but include infection or tearing out of the sutures, as well as inadvertent suture placement through the bladder wall. Voiding difficulties may occur postoperatively as a result of the increased outflow resistance, and late failure of the procedure due to tearing or fracture of the sutures is well recognized.

Sling operations are among the combined vaginal and suprapubic procedures (though they may employ a single approach) and are indicated for more complex, recurrent incontinence rather than as a primary procedure. Their complication rates are high, including significant voiding difficulties postoperatively as well as infection, haemorrhage and technical failure. Sling operations are useful when the urethra is scarred or the vagina stenosed but should not be thought of as first-line management for genuine stress incontinence.

Abdominal procedures are many and varied. Marshall, Marchetti and Krantz (Marshall *et al.* 1949) first described the procedure which takes their name in a 54-year-old man who had developed stress incontinence following an abdomino-perineal excision of rectum. The operation is indicated for primary or recurrent stress incontinence not associated with anterior vaginal wall prolapse. After exposure of the bladder neck a nonabsorbable suture is used to hitch it up to the periosteum behind the symphysis pubis, with or without a preliminary urethral lengthening procedure. A success rate of 96% in nearly 4,000 patients has been reported by Krantz (1986) but not without complications. Some series report up to 5% incidence of osteitis pubis (probably due to periosteal infection following needle passage). Other problems include inadvertent bladder or urethral injury, failure of retention of the sutures to the back of the pubis and haemorrhage from the perivesical venous plexus.

Burch (1961) initially described a urethrovaginal fixation and then a urethrovesical suspension for the correction of stress incontinence. It has been modified by many surgeons but still has the original steps. The procedure achieves both bladder-neck and bladder-base elevation through suturing the paravaginal tissue in the lateral fornices to the ipsilateral ileopectineal ligament on either side. It is suitable for primary and recurrent stress incontinence, with or without anterior vaginal wall prolapse. Objective cure rates around 80% are generally reported, with greater success in patients for whom this is a primary procedure. Complications again include inadvertent injury to the bladder or urethra and haemorrhage from the perivesical veins. The incidence of urinary tract infection can be lowered by the use of suprapubic bladder drainage, but the late complications of voiding difficulties and detrusor instability are well recognized. Causes of failure with this technique include inability to elevate the bladder neck adequately, persistent or worsening detrusor instability and fibrosis of the urethral or paraurethral tissues. In spite of this, it remains the operation of choice for genuine stress incontinence with many surgeons, and it has been shown to have better long-term results when compared with both colposuspension or modified needle suspension (Bergman *et al.* 1989). It comes nearer the ideal 'best operation', for patients suitable for general anaesthetic, than the other procedures described, but it still involves a considerable peri- and postoperative morbidity as well as the need to remain in hospital for 5–7 days postoperatively.

Laparoscopic colposuspension embodies the principle of bladder-neck and bladder-base elevation but is achieved without the need for a traditional abdominal incision. It is an example of the many laparoscopic procedures that have demonstrated an evolutionary process with regard to technique. Early pioneers created a pneumoperitoneum and then incised the peritoneum above the bladder to gain access to the peritoneal space (Albala *et al.* 1992). Chapple (Chapple & Osborne 1992) has quite clearly shown that a direct retropubic insufflation is feasible, quicker and associated with less trauma. The ideal laparoscopic colposuspension must be as minimally invasive as the endoscopic Stamey bladder-neck suspension but have the same long-term results as an open Burch colposuspension.

Laparoscopic instrumentation

1 High-flow carbon dioxide insufflator
2 CCD camera and monitor
3 Veress needle (safety type)
4 0° 10mm laparoscope
5 One 10mm port and two 5mm ports with grips and converters/downsizers
6 Laparoscopic scissors (diathermy connection)
7 Laparoscopic dissecting forceps
8 Stamey bladder-neck suspension needle

Technique

1 The patient is placed in the lithotomy position with a 20–25° head-down tilt. The patient is prepared and draped to allow a synchronous pelvic laparoscopy and vaginal procedure to be carried out. A urethral catheter is used until all of the ports have been inserted.
2 A monitor should be placed at the foot of the table opposite the main operator who will probably stand on the left-hand side of the patient if he or she is right-handed (Fig. 16.1).
3 A small incision is made immediately above the symphysis pubis

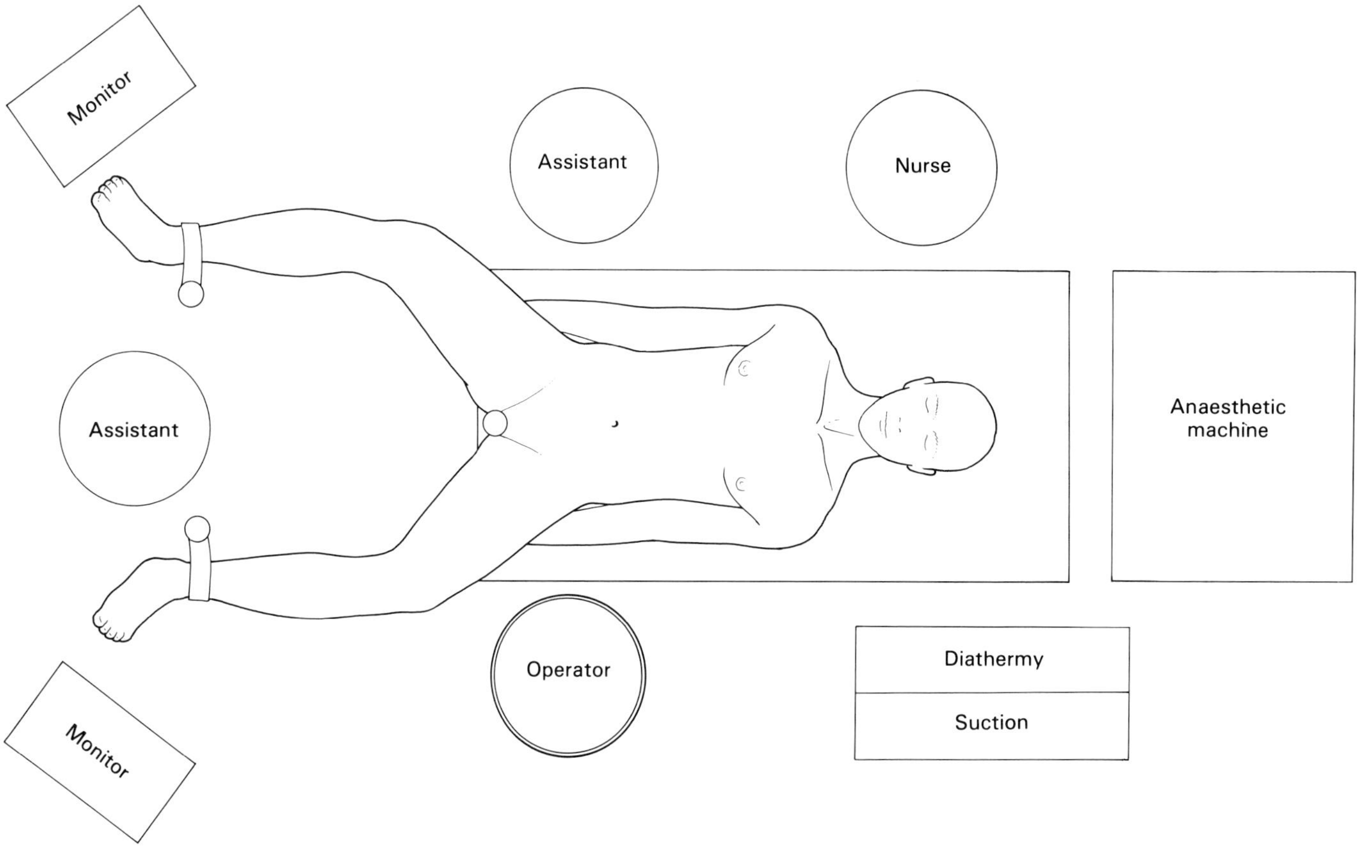

Fig. 16.1 The layout of the operating theatre equipment for a laparoscopic colposuspension.

and the Veress needle is inserted into the retropubic space. The operator must feel the symphysis with the tip of the needle to prevent inadvertent entry of the peritoneum. Carbon dioxide is insufflated to a volume of approximately 1–1.5 litres. The pressures will initially be quite high, which is in contrast to insufflation of the peritoneal cavity. As the peritoneal lining is stripped upwards, the tension and concomitant pressure falls to the normal range.

4 A 10mm port for the telescope is inserted at the site of the Veress needle, again keeping close to the symphysis pubis. Visual confirmation of being in the retropubic space is gained with the laparoscope. Two secondary 5mm ports are placed proximally and lateral to the telescope port as close to the edge of the rectus sheath as is possible to avoid epigastric artery injury. These ports are for the manipulative instruments (Fig. 16.2).

5 The fatty tissue lying across the bladder neck must be swept aside and care must be taken, because it often contains numerous veins. It is best to use soft dissecting instruments with the additional help of a finger in the vagina beneath the area of dissection. The paravaginal tissues are cleared adjacent to the bladder neck.

6 The colposuspension itself should ideally be created with three 1/0 silk sutures on either side with knots tied intra- or extracorporeally.

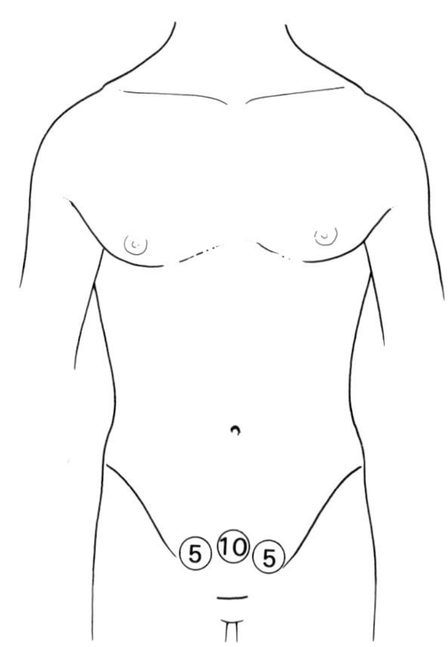

Fig. 16.2 The port sites for a laparoscopic colposuspension.

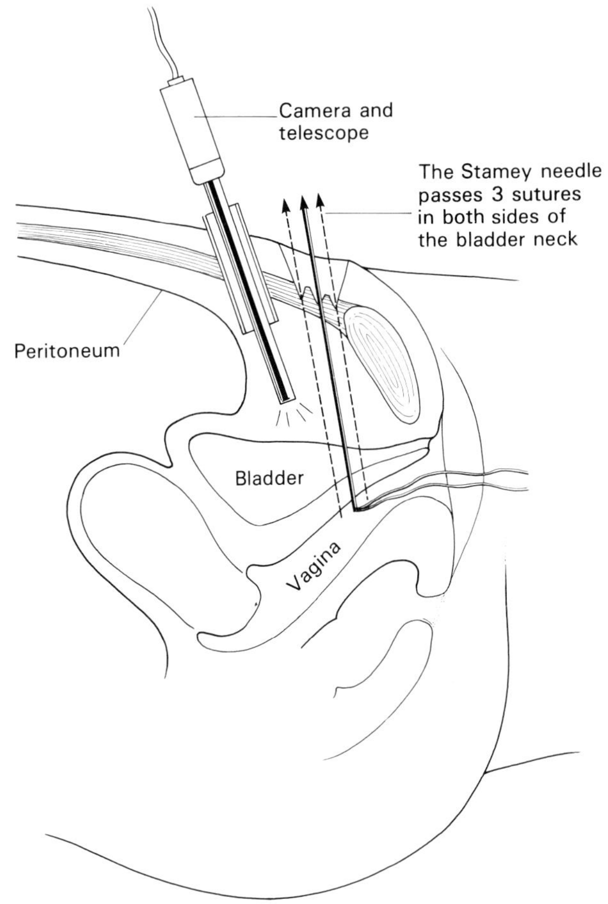

Fig. 16.3 The Stamey needle is passed three times on each side up laparoscopic vision, and the sutures are tied above the rectus sheath as described by Chapple.

However, we have found that the space and elasticity of some patients' tissues do not allow reasonable placement of these sutures and in these cases the modified Stamey procedure of Chapple is recommended. This involves passage of a nylon suture by means of a Stamey needle through the vagina as in its open counterpart but guiding this under direct vision through the retropubic space and out onto the abdominal wall (Fig. 16.3). A minimum of two sutures can then be placed on either side and tied above the rectus sheath. Correct placement of all sutures should be checked with a cystoscope at the end of the procedure.

7 The ports are removed under direct vision and the carbon dioxide gas evacuated. A drain is not required.

8 The 10mm wound requires a fascial suture. Skin can be approximated with either steristrips or a 3/0 Ethylon suture. A urethral catheter is left in place for five days, but the patient can usually be discharged on the first postoperative day.

Discussion

Chapple (Chapple & Osborne 1992) has already presented preliminary results and although there were some failures in the first 15 cases, these were all due to technical problems before refinement of technique. Once successfully completed, the laparoscopic colposuspension seems to have produced good results comparable to that of an open Burch colposuspension. We have modified Chapple's technique, in those patients with a broad enough pelvis and lax enough paravaginal tissues to avoid the need for percutaneous suture placement, by using intracorporeal sutures. Our attempts to use staples have been disappointing because the tension of the joined tissues is too great.

References

Albala D.M., Schuessler W.W., Vancaille T.G. (1992) Laparoscopic bladder neck suspension. *Journal of Endourology*, **6**: 2, 137–41.

Bergman A., Koonings P.P., Ballard C.A. (1989) Primary stress urinary incontinence and pelvic relaxation: Prospective randomized comparison of three different operations. *American Journal of Obstetrics and Gynaecology*, **91**, 46–55.

Burch J.C. (1961) Urethrovaginal fixation to Cooper's ligament for correction of stress incontinence, cystocele and prolapse. *American Journal of Obstetrics and Gynecology*, **81**, 281.

Cardozo L.D. & Cutner A. (1992) Surgical management of genuine stress incontinence. *Contemporary Revue of Obstetrics and Gynaecology*, **4**, 36–41.

Chapple C.R. & Osborne J.L. (1992) Laparoscopic colposuspension—a new procedure. *Journal of Urology*, **147**: 4, 267A.

Kirby R.S. & Whiteway J.E. (1989) Results of Stamey bladder-neck suspension. *British Journal of Urology*, **63**, 21–33.

Krantz K.E. (1986) The Marshall-Marchetti-Krantz procedure. In *Surgery of female incontinence* (eds S.L. Stanton & T. Tanago), 2nd edn, pp. 87–93, Springer-Verlag, New York.

Marshall V.T., Marchetti A.A., Krantz K.E. (1949) The correction of stress incontinence by simple vesico-urethral suspension. *Surgery, Gynaecology and Obstetrics*, **88**, 509–18.

Mundy A.R. (1983) A trial comparing the Stamey bladder neck procedure with colposuspension for the treatment of stress incontinence. *British Journal of Urology*, **55**, 687–90.

Pereyra A.J. (1959) A simplified surgical procedure for the correction of stress incontinence in women. *Western Journal of Surgery*, **67**, 223–6.

Weil A., Reves H., Bischoff P., Rottenberg R.D., Krauer I. (1984) Modifications of the urethral resting and stress profiles after different types of surgery for urinary stress incontinence. *British Journal of Obstetrics and Gynaecology*, **91**, 46–55.

17: Laparoscopic Bladder-Dome Transection

P. CARTER AND M.J. COPTCOAT

Introduction

The severely disabling symptoms associated with intractable detrusor instability have prompted continued exploration of surgical possibilities for those patients in whom bladder retraining and drug therapy have failed. Clam cystoplasty is practised by many surgeons with considerable success but is highly invasive, with a level of postoperative morbidity that makes it far from ideal as a procedure for curing or improving incontinence. Similarly, the results of sacral and parasacral parasympathectomy were very poor and did not justify the operative morbidity.

Since its introduction by Turner-Warwick and Ashken in 1967, modified open bladder transection has been used by many authors in the treatment of urge incontinence associated with detrusor instability and for nocturnal enuresis (Gibbon *et al.* 1973, Essenhigh & Yeates 1973, Hindmarsh *et al.* 1977, Janknegt *et al.* 1979, Mundy 1980). Accumulated success rates for the procedure were reported as approximately 75% but obvious disadvantages include the need for an abdominal incision and its associated morbidity as well as the significant number of patients who will receive no benefit from it. Many of the commonly reported complications stem from the need to completely transect the bladder wall; they include prolonged haematuria and suprapubic leakage, as well as urinary-tract infection.

The rationale for the procedure was based on the knowledge that nerve fibres supplying the detrusor enter the bladder at the level of the inferior vesical pedicle and spread upwards. Circumferential division of the bladder above the level of the ureters would disrupt the supply to the detrusor while leaving the sensory supply to the bladder base intact (Essenhigh & Yeates 1973). However, urodynamic testing and experimental studies in many patients reporting significant improvement following the procedure have failed to substantiate this theory.

Staskin *et al.* (1981) showed that a complete disruption of the anatomical and myoelectrical conductivity of the detrusor functional syncytium could be achieved by transection. They were also able to show that disruption of the intramural neurones led to complete adrenergic denervation of the detrusor as well as partial cholinergic decentralization in their beagle experimental model.

Although the similarity between dog and human detrusor is not exact, Parsons *et al.* (1984) used Staskin's beagle model to justify their technique of endoscopic bladder transection, postulating that the benefits from open or endoscopic transection should be similar.They were able to show a similar symptomatic improvement to that seen with open surgery but achieved it with considerably lower morbidity. The technique involved a circumferential transection 2cm above the trigone anteriorly to 2cm above the bladder neck. Mucosa and muscle were incised down to extra vesical fat, insuring that all detrusor fibres were cut.

Extravasation and haemorrhage were reported as minimal with very few other side effects. Follow-up showed a markedly similar outcome to that of patients undergoing open surgery, with over 80% of patients achieving an excellent or satisfactory outcome. Longer-term follow-up, as with open surgery, showed a recurrence of symptoms in 10% of patients but also showed that some patients achieved benefit as late as six months postoperatively.

Whether because of difficulties involved in visualizing the transection course and depth or because of the complications of haemorrhage and extravasation, the procedure failed to become widely accepted and now appears to be little used.

An operative laparoscopic technique is possible that achieves a transection on the 'correct' side of the bladder is technically easy and has a lower morbidity. Laparoscopic bladder-dome transection offers the advantage of a precise 'disruption' of the detrusor functional syncytium (as well as limited intramural neuronal division) but keeps the mucosa intact, so reducing the complications of haemorrhage, extravasation and sepsis.

Laparoscopic instrumentation

1 High-flow carbon dioxide insufflator
2 CCD camera and at least one monitor
3 Veress needle (safety)
4 0° 10mm laparoscope (30° optional)
5 Three 10mm ports with grips and converters/downsizers
6 Laparoscopic curved microscissors (diathermy connection)
7 Laparoscopic soft grasping forceps
8 Laparoscopic curved dissecting forceps
9 Endoclip* Applier (small)

Technique

1 Under a general anaesthetic with muscle paralysis and assisted ventilation, the patient is put in a supine position with a 20–25° head-down tilt. The laparoscopy should be preceded by a cystoscopy. A

*A trademark of the United States Surgical Corporation (AutoSuture).

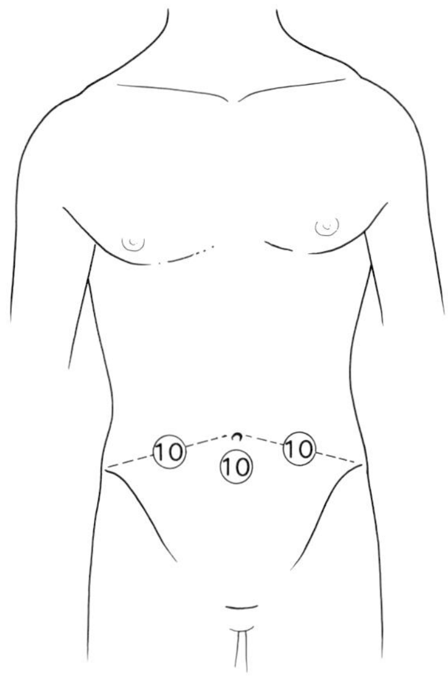

Fig. 17.1 Sites of the three 10mm ports for a laparoscopic bladder transection.

urethral catheter is left in situ and connected to a bag of saline so that a constant 200–300ml can be infused and kept in the bladder during the bladder transection, *after* insertion of the ports. Hip flexion is not required.

2 Formation of the pneumoperitoneum: the Veress needle is inserted at an angle of 45° into the empty pelvis. The position should be checked by aspiration and infusion of 5ml of saline, and the intra-abdominal pressure should remain below 12ml of mercury during insufflation. In the hands of inexperienced laparoscopists, disposable Veress needles with a safety shield are safer. Previous major abdominal surgery is a relative contraindication. A previous appendicectomy is unlikely to have produced difficult intra-abdominal adhesions but anything more significant than this may produce an unnecessarily difficult procedure out of proportion to the open alternatives for a bladder transection.

The Veress needle should be inserted through a subumbilical incision in an unscarred abdomen but in the presence of an appendicectomy scar, it is wise either to insert the Veress needle at the lateral edge of the left rectus sheath, where one of the secondary ports would normally be placed, or to introduce the first port with a Hasson cut-down technique in this lateral position.

3 Three 10mm ports are placed according to the diagram (Fig. 17.1). The subumbilical port is used for the telescope. The two secondary ports along the lateral edges of the rectus sheath are for manipulative and dissecting instruments. The use of two 10mm ports allows the Endoclip Applier to be introduced through either of them. The ports should be fixed with either grips or purse-string sutures.

4 The operator stands on the contralateral side of the patient whilst the camera-holder stands on the ipsilateral side (as in Fig. 11.2).

5 The video monitors should be at the bottom corners of the operating table.

6 Dissection is required on each side of the bladder so that the ultimate serosal incision can extend as far as possible. This will require division of the superior vesical pedicle between double clips. A coronal serosal incision is then made with the tip of the scissors using diathermy. The blunt tip of the scissors prevents inadvertent penetration of the mucosa. Incision is taken down until the blue coloured mucosa bulges through the serosa (Fig. 17.2).

7 A Silastic 16F urethral catheter is left indwelling for two weeks but the patient can usually be managed as a day case.

8 The ports must be removed under direct vision. All carbon dioxide is evacuated.

9 To prevent wound-herniation, all wounds require a deep fascial suture. The skin can either be sutured with a subcuticular absorbable suture or steristripped. Patients require two to three hours to recover and can then be discharged home.

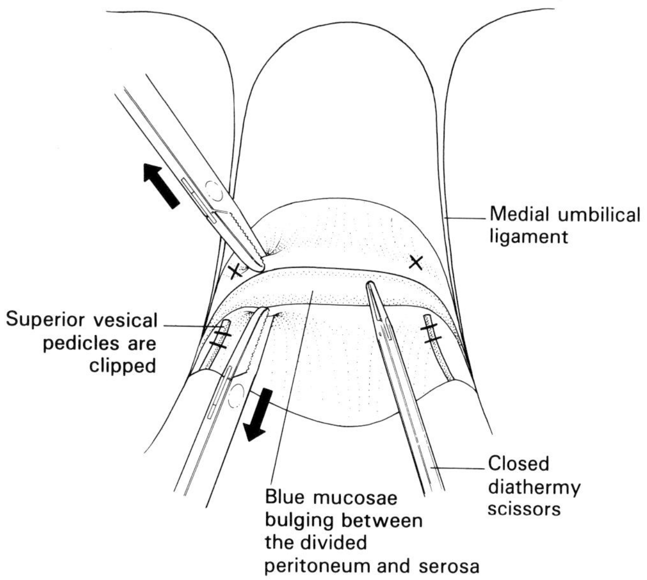

Fig. 17.2 The superior vesical pedicles are divided between clips. A coronal incision is made in the peritoneum and bladder serosa with a combination of diathermy and sharp dissection.

Discussion

One of my constant themes in this book has been to identify new techniques that can be employed because of laparoscopy rather than simply as an attempt to reproduce open operations with minimal access. The laparoscopic bladder-dome transection is an example of this in that it is a technique which would not have been previously employed but achieves a result that is anatomically and physiologically more consistent with the hypothesis of why a bladder transection should work for bladder instability.

All but one of our cases has been managed in our day-case centre. There have been no complications and we await the long-term evaluation of our results with interest. In the short term, there has been a 60% complete response and 40% partial response with regard to symptoms of urgency, urge incontinence and frequency. It has been difficult to further assess these results with urodynamics because many of our patients have presented to us with a history suggestive of primary bladder instability but without urodynamic evidence. Such a minimally invasive procedure as the laparoscopic bladder-dome transection seems to be a very reasonable surgical alternative when medical therapy has failed.

References

Essenhigh D.M. & Yeates W.K. (1973) Transection of the bladder with particular reference to enuresis. *British Journal of Urology*, **45**, 299–305.

Gibbon N.O.K., Jameson R.M., Heal M.R., Abel B.J. (1973) Transection of the bladder for adult enuresis and allied conditions. *British Journal of Urology*, **45**, 306–9.

Hindmarsh J.R., Essenhigh D.M., Yeates W.K. (1977) Bladder transection for adult enuresis. *British Journal of Urology*, **49**, 515–21.

Janknegt R.A., Moonen W.A., Schreinemachers L.M.H. (1979) Transection of the bladder as a method of treatment in adult enuresis nocturna. *British Journal of Urology*, **51**, 275–7.

Mundy A.R. (1980) Bladder transection for urge incontinence associated with detrusor instability. *British Journal of Urology*, **52**, 480–3.

Parsons K.F., Machin D.G., Woolfenden K.A., Walmsley B., Abercrombie G.F., Vinnicombe J. (1984) Endoscopic bladder transection. *British Journal of Urology*, **56**, 625–8.

Staskin D.R., Parsons K.F., Levin R.M., Wein A.J. (1981) Bladder transection—a functional, neurophysical, neuropharmacological and neuroanatomical study. *British Journal of Urology*, **53**, 552–7.

Turner-Warwick R.T. & Ashken M.H. (1967) The functional results of partial, subtotal and total cystoplasty, with special reference to ureterocaecocystoplasty, selective sphincterotomy and cystocystoplasty. *British Journal of Urology*, **39**, 3–12.

18: Laparoscopic Ileal Conduit Diversion

M.J. COPTCOAT AND A.D. JOYCE

Introduction

Since 1950, the ileal conduit described by Bricker has been by far the most common type of supravesical urinary diversion, and there have been only a few surgical modifications to his ureteral reimplantation into the ileal segment. Most patients who receive an ileal loop have concomitant open surgical removal of their bladders and other pelvic organs for cancer. At this point in the development of laparoscopic surgery, a laparoscopic cystectomy is feasible but not refined enough to become part of our surgical armamenterium. The type of patient who would benefit from a laparoscopic ileal loop conduit would thus be a patient with a benign bladder and intractable voiding problems, such as a patient with a neuropathic bladder.

Laparoscopic instrumentation

1 High-flow carbon dioxide insufflator
2 CCD camera and at least one monitor
3 Veress needle (safety)
4 0° 10mm laparoscope (30° optional)
5 0° 5mm laparoscope
6 One 10mm port, two 12mm ports and three 5mm ports with grips and converters/downsizers
7 Laparoscopic curved scissors (diathermy connection)
8 Laparoscopic soft bowel-grasping forceps (x 2)
9 Laparoscopic curved dissecting forceps
10 Laparoscopic Babcock forceps
11 Endoclip* Applier (medium/large)
12 Endo GIA* 30 stapler

Technique

1 A preliminary cystoscopy and insertion of bilateral self-retaining ureteric stents is undertaken. Each ureteric orifice is then circumcised with a diathermy knife under direct vision. This will facilitate an easy uretero-vesical division during later laparoscopic dissection, and it will also provide the maximum length of ureter (see point 8 below).

*A trademark of the United States Surgical Corporation (AutoSuture).

2 Under a general anaesthetic with muscle paralysis and assisted ventilation, the patient is placed in the supine position with a 20–25° head-down tilt. Urethral catheterization is required.

3 Formation of the pneumoperitoneum: the Veress needle is inserted at an angle of 45° into the empty pelvis. The position should be checked by aspiration and infusion of 5ml of saline, and the intra-abdominal pressure should remain below 12ml of mercury during insufflation. In the hands of inexperienced laparoscopists, disposable Veress needles with a safety shield are safer. Previous major abdominal surgery is a relative contraindication. Adhesions will have to be taken down carefully under direct vision.

The Veress needle should be inserted through a subumbilical incision in an unscarred abdomen but in the presence of an appendicectomy scar, it is wise either to insert the Veress needle at the lateral edge of the left rectus sheath, where one of the secondary ports would normally be placed, or to introduce the first port with a Hasson cut-down technique in this lateral position.

4 The ports are placed according to the diagram (Fig. 18.1). The subumbilical port is for the 10mm telescope. The two 12mm ports are the best to use for primary dissecting and manipulative instrumentation, and the more laterally placed 5mm ports can be used for grasping instruments held by an assistant. The midline 5mm port is for the introduction of the 5mm telescope with its own light source for appropriate background highlighting of omental vessels. The ports should be fixed with either grips or purse-string sutures.

5 The operator stands on the left side of the patient and will require a camera-holder on the opposite side and a second assistant on his own side (as in Fig. 13.2).

6 Monitors should be at the bottom corners of the operating table.

7 After inspection of the abdominal contents, the small bowel is removed from the pelvis. The peritoneal reflections lateral to the caecum and sigmoid colon are divided to allow identification of the ureters as they cross into the pelvis. The ureters are dissected down to the bladder and, with gentle traction, freed from their insertion into the bladder. The ureteric stents should then be lying free within the abdomen (Fig. 18.2).

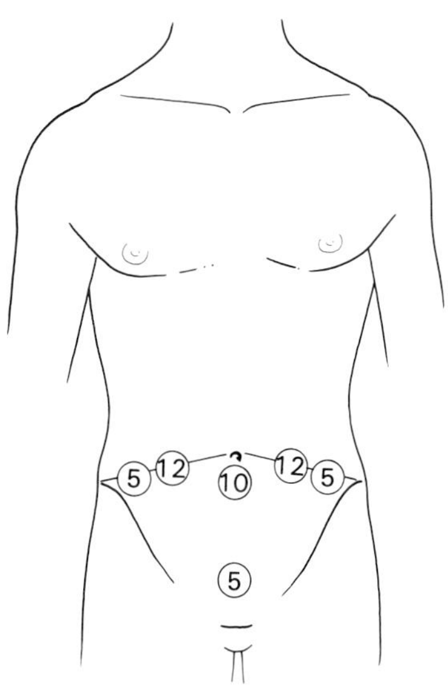

Fig. 18.1 Sites for one 10mm, two 12mm and three 5mm ports for a laparoscopic ileal conduit.

8 Approximately 15cm of small bowel are identified at least 20cm proximal to the ileosigmoid junction. The bowel can be initially held up with soft grasping forceps but it should then be held with sutures placed percutaneously, taken through the wall of the bowel and then back out again close their point of entry. This is achieved with a 1/0 coloured monofilament suture and straight needle. A third hanging suture is also required at the midpoint of the selected ileal segment to provide a better exposure of the mesenteric vessels.

A 5mm telescope and separate light source are used to provide background lighting of the mesenteric vessels. The mesentery is

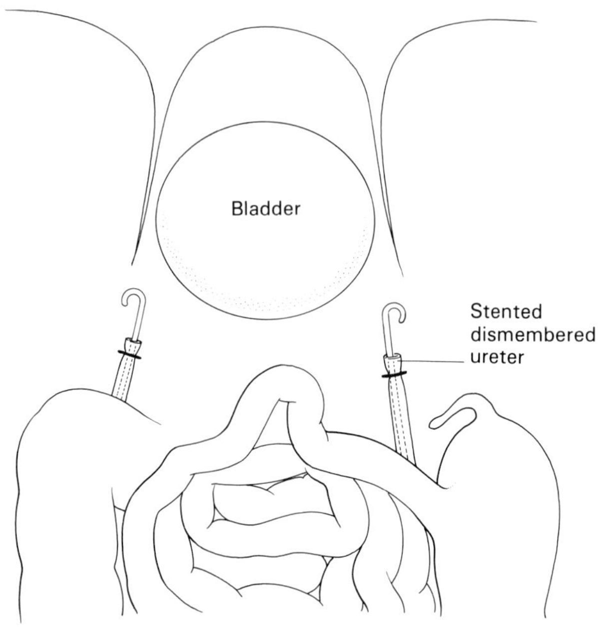

Fig. 18.2 The peritoneum is incised to reveal both ureters, which are dissected down to the bladder and then pulled through with their stents, following a preliminary transurethral circumcision of each uretic orifice.

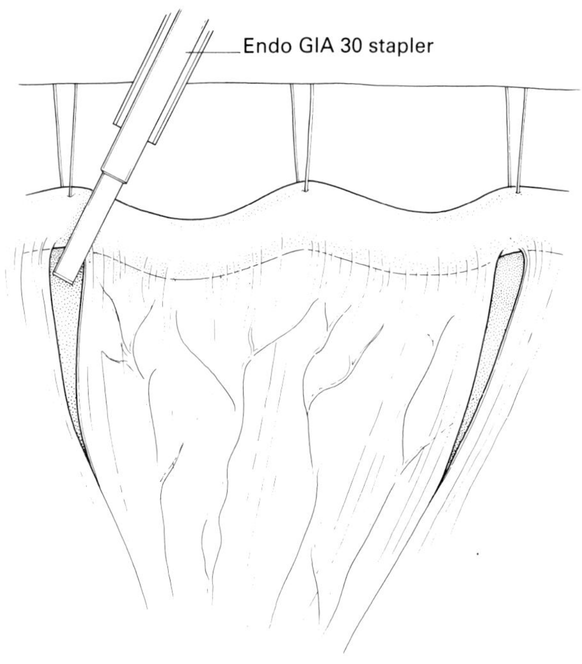

Fig. 18.3 The ileum is held up with three holding sutures to the abdominal wall. The mesentery is divided, with the vascular Endo GIA 60 stapler, before dividing the ileum itself with bowel staples.

perforated on both sides towards the apex of the pedicle. The Endo GIA 30 stapler is then placed across the bowel just inside each holding suture (Fig. 18.3). This divides the bowel between the stapled ends. Further use of the Endo GIA 30 stapler will then take the division down to the perforations that have been made towards the apex of the pedicle.

A 15cm length of ileum with closed ends should now be viable on its own pedicle. Reanastomosis of the ileum is brought about by

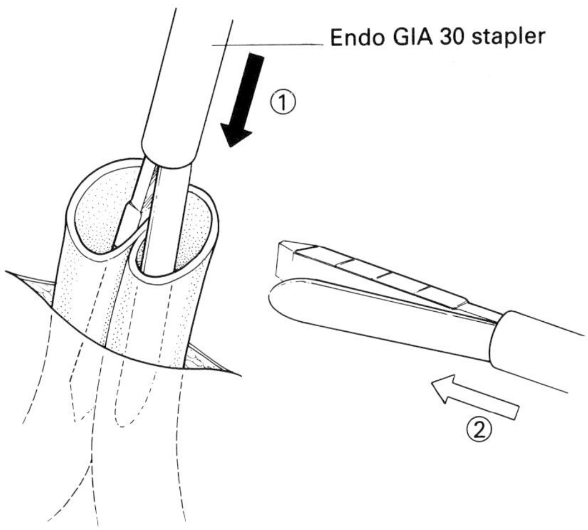

Fig. 18.4 The Endo GIA 30 stapler is used extracorporeally to create a side to side small-bowel anastomosis, after delivering the ends through the 16mm port site

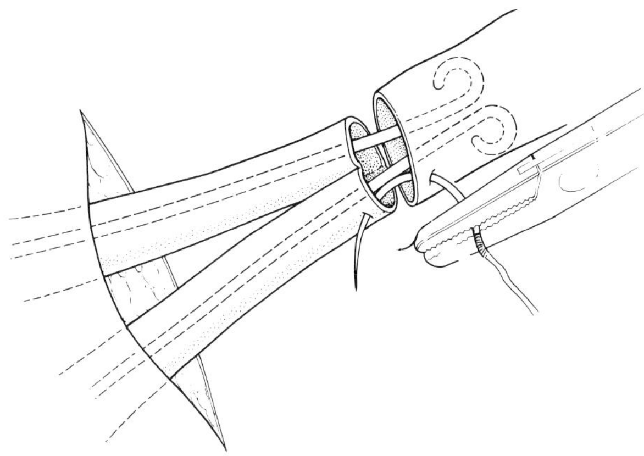

Fig. 18.5 The extra length of the ureters allows the uretero-ileal anastomosis to be created extracorporeally.

detaching the holding sutures and bringing the bowel ends side by side with the use of the Babcock forceps. A 2/0 suture is used to stabilize the anti-mesenteric border of the ileum 6–7cm from the site of reanastomosis.

A bowel anastomosis is quite feasible within the abdomen but the mesentery is usually long enough to allow the two ends to be brought out through one of the 12mm port sites. The Endo GIA 30 stapler can then be used much more easily outside of the body under direct vision to create a side to side anastomosis (Fig. 18.4). Sometimes the 12mm port site needs a further 1cm enlargement and this will have to be subsequently countered with a purse-string suture when further laparoscopic dissection continues upon reintroduction of the port.

The uretero-ileal anastomosis can again take place within the abdomen, using a continuous laparoscopic suturing technique, but it is far less time-consuming again to bring this out onto the surface (Fig. 18.5). The maximum ureteric length gained by carrying out an initial transurethral ureteric resection facilitates this. A routine

Wallis anastomosis can be performed using either catgut or vicryl or Polysorb suture. The ureteric stents are left in situ. This anastomosis is allowed to drop back into the abdomen and after a final check for adequate haemostasis, the ileal stoma can be created in a routine fashion with an everted nipple.

9 Two 10mm drains are placed in the pelvis. One is guided to the site of bowel anastomosis and the second to the uretero-ileal anastomosis under direct vision.

10 The ports must be removed under direct vision. All carbon dioxide is evacuated.

11 To prevent wound-herniation, all wounds require a deep fascial suture. The skin can either be sutured with a subcuticular absorbable suture or steristripped. Patients require two to three hours to recover and can then be discharged home.

Discussion

Kozminski & Partamian (1992) were the first to report a laparoscopic ileal loop conduit technique, and our method varies only slightly. They too realized the potential for intracorporeal anastomosis of both bowel and ureter to bowel, but with present stapling instrumentation and suture methods extracorporeal anastomosis makes the procedure much more rapid and possibly safer. The laparoscopic ileal conduit is the first of many types of supravesical diversion that can probably be undertaken in a much more minimally invasive way, and their development will go hand in hand with the refinement of the laparoscopic cystectomy, so that such surgery can be available for our patients with bladder cancer.

References

Bricker E.M. (1950) Bladder substitution after pelvic evisceration. *Surgical Clinics of North America*, **30**, 1511.

Kozminski M. & Partamian K.O. (1992) Case report of laparoscopic ileal loop conduit. *Journal of Endourology*, **6**: 2, 147–50.

19: Laparoscopic Partial Cystectomy

M. J. COPTCOAT

Introduction

Advances made in laparoscopic surgery during recent years have made it possible to perform almost any procedure. A total cystectomy has been described by Parra *et al.* (1992). At the present time, however, a sense of proportion must be exercised, and whilst a total cystectomy is quite feasible, it is clear that still some improvement in instrumentation is required to allow easy dissection and stapling of the inferior vesical pedicles. This will follow shortly but in the meantime, the laparoscopic partial cystectomy is a very straightforward procedure. There are many fewer indications for a partial cystectomy, but it has achieved its greatest success as an open procedure in the treatment of highly localized superficial bladder cancer. Indications for a segmental or partial cystectomy include the histologically well-documented presence of a solitary neoplasm at least 3 cm distant from the bladder neck, inaccessibility of a lesion to transurethral resection or location of tumour in a vesical diverticulum. Contraindications include recurrent or multiple tumours, the presence of flat carcinoma in situ, involvement of the bladder neck in women or invasion of the prostatic urethra in men, extravesical extensive disease, prior irradiation and inadequate bladder volume. If a partial cystectomy is undertaken, tumour spill must be avoided and a cystotomy should be done as far away from the tumour as possible. Precise mucosal apposition closure is probably also important, so that any abnormal mucosa is not inadvertently buried in the bladder wall. Theoretically, suprapubic catheter drainage may permit extravesical seeding of tumour, though there are no case reports.

Laparoscopic instrumentation

1 High-flow carbon dioxide insufflator
2 CCD camera and at least one monitor
3 Veress needle (safety)
4 0° 10 mm laparoscope (30° optional)
5 One 10 mm port, two 12 mm ports and two 5 mm ports with grips and converters/downsizers
6 Laparoscopic curved scissors (diathermy connection)
7 Laparoscopic soft grasping forceps (x two)
8 Laparoscopic curved dissecting forceps
9 Laparoscopic Babcock forceps

10 Endoclip* Applier (medium/large)
11 Endo GIA* 30 stapler

Technique

1 Under a general anaesthetic with muscle paralysis and assisted ventilation, the patient is placed in the supine position with a 20–25° head-down tilt. A large calibre (18 or 20F) catheter is required.
2 Formation of the pneumoperitoneum: the Veress needle is inserted just lateral to the umbilicus at an angle of 45° into the empty pelvis. The position should be checked by aspiration and infusion of 5ml of saline, and the intra-abdominal pressure should remain below 12ml of mercury during insufflation. In the hands of inexperienced laparoscopists, disposable Veress needles with a safety shield are safer. Previous major abdominal surgery is a relative contraindication. A previous appendicectomy is unlikely to have produced difficult intra-abdominal adhesions but anything more significant than this may produce an unnecessarily difficult procedure out of proportion to the open alternatives for a partial cystectomy.
3 The ports are placed according to the diagram (Fig. 19.1). The routine subumbilical port is not used in this case, nor are any lower midline ports because of the possibility of penetration through an involved urachal remnant. The Veress needle and subsequent telescope ports are inserted just lateral to the umbilicus. The secondary 12mm ports along the lateral edges of the rectus sheath are for manipulative and dissecting instruments, and the more laterally placed 5mm ports can be used by an assistant either for retraction or for grasping.
4 The operator stands on the left side of the patient and will require a camera-holder on the opposite side and a second assistant on his own side (Fig 12.2).
5 The video monitors should be at the bottom corners of the operating table.
6 After inspection of the entire abdominal contents for possible metastatic spread when indicated, the small bowel and adherent sigmoid colon should be manipulated free from the pelvis. The peritoneum should be incised over the dome of the bladder. The superior vesical pedicles should be divided between double clips or, if there is difficulty in identifying the vessels, the Endo GIA 30 stapler should be used. Stay sutures into the bladder add stability during subsequent partial cystectomy, and these are best introduced percutaneously as separate hanging sutures using a 1/0 coloured monofilament suture on a straight needle. The appropriate part of the bladder is resected and placed into an organ entrapment bag prior to removal through

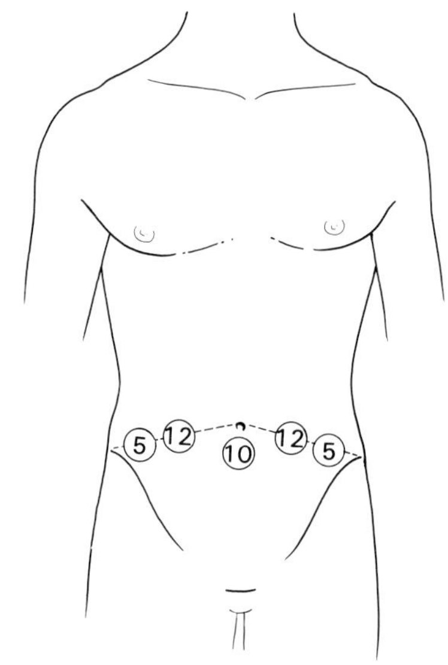

Fig. 19.1 Sites for one 10mm, two 12mm and two 5mm ports for a laparoscopic partial cystectomy.

*A trademark of the United States Surgical Corporation (AutoSuture).

one of the 12 mm ports, which usually require slight enlargement by an extra 0.5–1 cm. Removal of the organ bag should be left until after resuturing of the bladder edges to preserve the efficient pneumoperitoneum. The bladder can be closed in one layer with a continuous 2/0 absorbable suture.

7 A drain is guided down into either side of the pelvis under direct vision and left in situ for 48 hours.

8 The ports must be removed under direct vision. All carbon dioxide is evacuated.

9 To prevent wound-herniation, all wounds require a deep fascial suture. The skin can either be sutured with a subcuticular absorbable suture or steristripped. Patients require two to three hours to recover and can usually be discharged after three to four days, with a urethral catheter that should be left in situ for three weeks.

Discussion

Our experience with the laparoscopic partial cystectomy is limited but all cases have been straightforward, with minimal blood loss and no requirement for transfusion. All patients were managed with a urethral catheter for three weeks, and normal voiding patterns returned within 4–6 months.

Das (1992) described the laparoscopic removal of a bladder diverticulum. This was by a transperitoneal approach. Diverticulae often open close to a ureteral orifice and in these cases, ureteric catheterization is recommended.

Future laparoscopic bladder techniques will probably involve both transurethral and synchronous laparoscopic transperitoneal procedures. This is an exciting area of development and will go hand in hand with our laparoscopic work on reconstruction.

References

Das S. (1992) Laparoscopic removal of bladder diverticulum. *Journal of Urology*, **148**, 1837–9.

Parra R.O., Andrus C.H., Jones J.P., Boullier J.A. (1992) Laparoscopic cystectomy: Initial report on a new treatment for the retained bladder. *Journal of Urology*, **148**, 1140–4.

20: Laparoscopic Lymphocele Drainage

M. J. COPTCOAT AND A. D. JOYCE

Introduction

Lymphoceles represent an extraperitoneal fluid collection in the transplant fossa from leak of lymphatic fluid in the post-transplant period. This is most often a consequence of inadequate ligature of divided lymphatics when the iliac vessels were skeletonized for the graft implantation.

Clinically, lymphoceles may compress the transplanted ureter or the iliac vein, with expected secondary manifestations, such as ureteral obstruction and oedema of the ipsilateral lower extremity. Diagnosis of a lymphocele can be confirmed by ultrasonography.

Treatment of small lymphoceles involves percutaneous drainage under ultrasound control, but this can lead to secondary infection and sometimes to persistence of the lymphocele. Permanent treatment, and certainly the first-line management of large lymphoceles, usually involves surgical intervention, with drainage of fluid and internal marsupialization of the lymphocele cavity into the peritoneal cavity by excision of perineum to create a peritoneal window for subsequent internal drainage of the fluid. Such a definitive procedure can also be carried out laparoscopically.

Laparoscopic instrumentation

1 High-flow carbon dioxide insufflator
2 CCD camera and at least one monitor
3 Veress needle (safety)
4 0° 10mm laparoscope (30° optional)
5 Three 10mm ports with grips and converters/downsizers
6 Laparoscopic curved microscissors (diathermy connection)
7 Laparoscopic soft grasping forceps
8 Laparoscopic curved dissecting forceps
9 Laparoscopic aspirator/irrigator

Technique

1 Under a general anaesthetic with muscle paralysis and assisted ventilation, the patient is put in a supine position with a 20–25° head-down tilt. A catheter is not usually required if the patient's bladder has recently emptied. Hip flexion is not required.

2 Formation of the pneumoperitoneum: the Veress needle is inserted

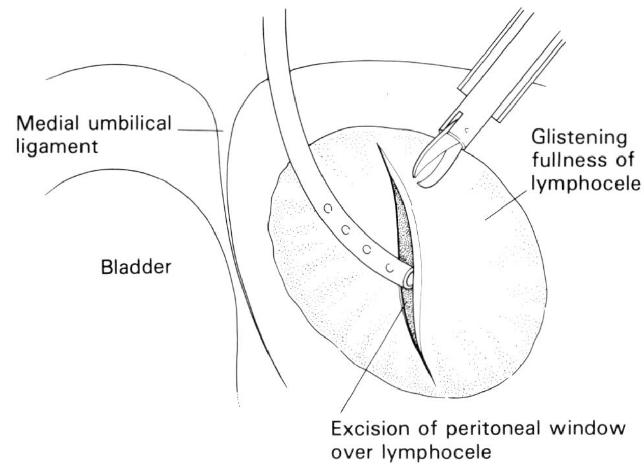

Fig. 20.1 The lymphocele is incised longitudinally under direct vision with scissors, and a drain is directed down into the peritoneal window.

at an angle of 45° into the empty pelvis. The position should be checked by aspiration and infusion of 5 ml of saline, and the intra-abdominal pressure should remain below 12 ml of mercury during insufflation. In the hands of inexperienced laparoscopists, the disposable Veress needles with a safety shield are safer. Previous major abdominal surgery is a relative contraindication. A previous appendicectomy is unlikely to have produced difficult intra-abdominal adhesions but anything more significant than this may produce an unnecessarily difficult procedure out of proportion to the open alternatives for a lymphocele drainage. The Veress needle should be inserted through a subumbilical incision in an unscarred abdomen but in the presence of an appendicectomy scar, it is wise either to insert the Veress needle at the lateral edge of the left rectus sheath, where one of the secondary ports would normally be placed, or to introduce the first port with a Hasson cut-down technique in this lateral position.

3 Three 10 mm ports are placed according to the diagram in Chapter 17 (Fig. 17.1). The subumbilical port is used for the telescope. The two secondary ports along the lateral edges of the rectus sheath are for manipulative and dissecting instruments. The use of two 10 mm ports allows the Endoclip Applier to be introduced through either of them. The ports should be fixed with either grips or purse-string sutures.

4 The operator stands on the contralateral side of the patient, whilst the camera-holder stands on the ipsilateral side (as in Fig. 11.2).

5 The video monitors should be at the bottom corners of the operating table.

6 The lymphocele is very obvious beneath the peritoneum, and it can be easily incised with the laparoscopic scissors. An aspirator should be held in the other hand, so that the contents can be immediately aspirated.

7 The drain is directed under vision down into the opened lymphocele and left for a further 48 hours (Fig. 20.1).

8 The ports must be removed under direct vision. All carbon dioxide is evacuated.
9 To prevent wound-herniation, all wounds require a deep fascial suture. The skin can either be sutured with a subcuticular absorbable suture or steristripped.

Discussion

Our attempts at laparoscopic transperitoneal lymphocele drainage have so far been successful in all cases without permanent marsupialization. This is probably due to the large incision in the back of the lymphocele, but the placement of a continuous suture between the two cavities would not be difficult if this opening was shown to close spontaneously before drainage had stopped. One is sometimes concerned about the site of the ureter during incision of the lymphocele, and for this reason, diathermy is not recommended. Our routine use of the laparoscopic scissors has been both precise and safe.

Index

Page numbers in **bold** refer to tables, those in *italic* to figures.